Midwifery Questions

Midwifery Questions Answered

Queen Charlotte's Hospital Midwifery Tutors
Edited by Valerie Smith

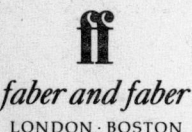

faber and faber
LONDON · BOSTON

First published in 1988
by Faber and Faber Limited
3 Queen Square London WC1N 3AU

Photoset by Parker Typesetting Service Leicester
Printed in Great Britain by
Cox & Wyman Ltd, Reading
All rights reserved

© V. Smith, L. Cornford-Wood, S. McDonald,
E. Davidson, J. Weston, L. Crooke and
M. Adams, 1988

*This book is sold subject to the condition that it
shall not, by way of trade or otherwise, be lent,
resold, hired out or otherwise circulated without the
publisher's prior consent in any form of binding or
cover other than that in which it is published and
without a similar condition including this condition
being imposed on the subsequent purchaser.*

British Library Cataloguing in Publication Data

Smith, Valerie
Midwifery questions answered.
1. Midwifery – Questions & answers
I. Title
610.73'678'076

ISBN 0-571-15051-9

Contents

	Foreword *Norma Naisbitt*	vii
	Preface	ix
1	Examinations and the midwifery profession *L. Cornford-Wood*	1
	History	1
	Why do we need examinations?	3
2	Studying for exams *S. McDonald, V. Smith*	6
	Physical and mental preparation	6
	Handwriting, spelling and presentation	9
	Other aids to learning	10
3	General principles of examination technique *E. Davidson*	12
	Types of question	12
	Paper and question planning	13
	Question construction	14
	Content	17
	Diagrams	18
	Timing	18
	Handwriting	19
	Final shopping day before the examination	20
	The day before the examination	20
	On entering the examination room	21

4	The viva voce *J. Weston*	22
	The examiner	23
	Overcoming nerves	24
	Trial runs	24
5	Weighting, marking and moderating *L. Crooke*	26
	Profile of the examiners	26
	Weighting	26
	The viva	28
	Marking	28
	Moderating	29
6	Midwifery qualifying examination: Differences in the examination system *M. Adams*	31
	England	31
	Scotland	32
	Northern Ireland	33
7	Advanced Diploma of Midwifery Examination *M. Adams*	34
	Midwifery and paediatrics	35
	Behavioural sciences	35
	The midwifery profession	35
8	Sample questions and answers	37
	Introduction	37
	Long questions	39
	Short questions	89
	Advanced Diploma in Midwifery questions	102
	Appendix: Past papers from the English National Board, Scottish National Board and Northern Ireland National Board	108

Foreword

Although the purpose and value of examinations continues to be debated there remains a strong belief that entry to a profession should be by a recognized examination. The key to the profession, however, should not be isolated from the course, neither should it take over the course or be the only assessment tool.

The course leading to registration as a midwife should be designed to prepare the student midwife to fulfil the role of a competent practitioner with the midwifery qualifying examination as the key to practice.

An examination should assess what is prescribed, do so clearly and in a meaningful way, thus allowing the candidate the best possible opportunity to demonstrate her cognitive skills, decision-making and attitudes.

This book, with detailed explanation of the format of the examination, explanation of the examination questions and guidance, should provide valuable assistance not only for those entering the midwifery qualifying examination but also for those who are assisting in the preparation of the future practitioner.

Norma Naisbitt
Education Officer
Midwifery Education, Training and Practice
English National Board

Preface

This book has been written in an attempt to illustrate the present-day midwifery examination system in the United Kingdom. Although midwifery education has changed considerably over the past ten to twenty years we are still faced, at present, with an examination at the end of training for which we need to prepare students.

An outline of the concepts of midwifery examinations, together with a general guide on the skills necessary for effective studying, is included to prepare students more fully for the final examination. This is followed by chapters on the general principles and preparation for the final examination plus an insight into what the examiner is looking for and how the content is assessed.

Differences in the examination system, administered by the National Boards for Nursing, Midwifery and Health Visiting, have been described, although the main text of the book relates to the English National Board examinations for England. The chapter on the Advanced Diploma of Midwifery has been included to encourage further study at a higher level and to give some guidance to those students undertaking this course.

The present examination for students aspiring to become Registered Midwives in England consists of two three-hour papers and a twenty-minute oral examination. The examination is designed to assess the student's competence to function as a safe practitioner of midwifery. To help students prepare for this role a section has been included with sample questions and appropriate answer plans in which our philosophy has been to move away from the model, prescriptive-type answer, towards giving guidelines as to what the answers should include. This is to encourage students to formulate individual answers while disciplining themselves to include all the relevant information in the time allowed.

Used properly, it is hoped that in addition to giving guidelines on studying and examination technique, the book will form a valuable revision source for the discerning student.

Unless indicated the questions are those from the examination papers set by the National Boards. The Appendix gives all papers set by the English, Scottish and Irish boards since the examinations were changed in 1986. We would like to extend to them our gratitude for allowing us to publish them in their entirety. Our particular thanks go to Miss Norma Naisbitt, Education Officer at the English National Board, for the advice and assistance with the content of the book and the assistance with the first part of Chapter 6 (England). Thanks also go to the many students who undertake midwifery training without whom this book would not be necessary.

Chapter 1

Examinations and the midwifery profession

HISTORY

The early history of the midwifery profession is well documented. Midwifery skills were traditionally passed on from mother to daughter. Nothing much changed until the nineteenth century when, in 1872, the Obstetrical Society of London established an examination – although it did not succeed in registering midwives.

In 1881 the Midwives Institute (now the Royal College of Midwives) was formed with the purpose of improving the status of midwives. The Institute recognizing that education would play a vital role in this.

It was not until 1902 that the first Midwives Act was passed – this was primarily for the protection of the public, but was also aimed at regulating midwifery practice and securing better training. Some of the power of the Central Midwives Board which was set up by the Act was to keep a Roll of Certified Midwives and to provide training and examinations to enable women to enter the Roll. Midwives whose names were first entered on the Roll were those who could prove that they had been in bona fide practice for at least a year prior to the Act and held the Diploma of the London Obstetrical Society or other recognized certificate. These women also had to be of good character – perhaps because of the primary function of the Act which was to protect the public from unworthy practitioners.

After 1 April 1910 unqualified persons were forbidden to attend women in childbirth except under the direction of a medical practitioner. Although many unqualified women could still practise, the basic tenet of qualification to practise was set. The 1921 Act strengthened control in midwifery, and finally the 1936 Midwives Act prohibited unqualified persons from practising midwifery.

The midwifery training course leading to enrolment/registration was originally of three months' duration (in 1902), expanding to twelve months by 1924. In 1938 training was divided into parts 1 and 2 with an examination after each part. Single-period training was reintroduced after 1968 and eighteen-month training was introduced in 1981 (in order to comply with EEC regulations).

With the passing of the Nurses, Midwives and Health Visitors Act 1979, the United Kingdom Central Council (UKCC) became responsible for the framing of midwifery practice, holding the Professional Register and, with the National Boards, responsible for regulating the examination system in accordance with the midwives' rules.

Historically practical and oral examinations formed an important part of the system, as did case histories and care studies. Recent changes have resulted in more account being taken of performance throughout the whole examination period (two three-hour papers and viva voce) rather than expecting the candidate to pass each specific part.

The trend for other parts of the Professional Register is to move towards devolved examinations (English National Board Circular, 1985) and there is a move to continuous assessment to remove some of the stress inherent in the examination system, and to provide a fairer system of evaluation. Whichever way the profession moves forward, some form of assessment will be used to allow candidates to register as midwives.

Examinations and the midwifery profession

WHY DO WE NEED EXAMINATIONS?

The rest of this chapter is concerned with summative assessments – the end examination. Whichever method of assessment is employed some value will be attributed to the student's work (clinical and theoretical), and therefore some level of attainment commented on.

Assessment is part of everyday life. We make decisions about people and situations and place our own values on what we perceive. In this sense assessment is a value judgement. During training assessments can be:

formative – during the learning programme
continuing – ongoing
summative – final assessment, an examination.

Why do we need to assess students?

It is a condition of midwifery, and indeed any other profession, that a value is placed on entry to that profession. An important part of examinations is the value that is placed on them, not only by the profession itself, but by the public at large. The examination is used as the measure of choosing the right and proper candidate to admit to the profession. It is seen as the gateway to professional practice. The public has a need for care to be given by competent practitioners. But the public cannot regulate the profession, an indication of who is or is not a member of that profession is needed. Passing a reliable examination followed by registration provides that indication, and gives a measure of who is 'safe' to practice. This is especially important within the context of independent practice.

The function of professional education is to provide learning opportunities to enable the student to gain sufficient knowledge, skills, and attitudes to enter the profession and therefore to practise. But as it is difficult to assess and measure these, how can we know that a student has the appropriate attributes? One way is the use of the examination system, wherein the level of competence and knowledge is measured. The examination also functions as an internal evaluation for the teaching and learning of midwifery, as standards are assessed by those already in the profession – student midwives are assessed by midwifery teachers, or mentor midwives.

The examination system must be valid when viewed from within the profession and by the public generally, who must be confident that the midwives produced are adequately trained and regulated.

Examinations must also be fair and reliable, and relevant to the actual work of the midwife. Questions now tend to be based on practical situations – a move away from straight anatomy and physiology with little relation to actual or potential problems.

Although in nurse training there is a move away from national standards, in midwifery a national qualifying standard is used to avoid variation in standards between midwifery schools, as marking by different assessors is bound to be somewhat subjective. Even if devolved and continuous assessment are used in the future, some standard measure of competency will have to be found.

Implicit in the examination system is that those who enter are considered fit to practise and enhance the profession. If this is not the case, then the system fails. Students who do not have the potential to practise at an acceptable standard should not be entered for examinations.

Certainly, no form of assessment covers all the ambiguities inherent in trying to assess a large number of potential midwives, but the examination system is a fair attempt.

Reference

English National Board circular (1985).
Examination Procedure for Courses in General Nursing Leading to Registration in Part 1 of the Register. ERDB, March.

Further reading

Bent, E. A. (1982). *The Growth and Development of Midwifery in Nursing, Midwifery and Health Visiting Since 1900,* eds Allen P. and Jolley M. Faber and Faber, London.

Jarvis, P. (1983). *Professional Education*. Croom Helm, Beckenham.

Jarvis, P. and Gibson, S. (1985). *The Teacher Practitioner in Nursing, Midwifery and Health Visiting*. Croom Helm, Beckenham.

Chapter 2
Studying for exams

PHYSICAL AND MENTAL PREPARATION

In order for a student to begin the necessary physical and psychological preparation for any examination it is essential that she is fully informed as early as possible following commencement of the course about factors pertaining to the examination. These should be the approximate time when the exams would be taken, the accepted format, and where copies of past examination papers can be obtained.

As the course develops the tutor organizes educational experiences for the students, including practical and written tests.

The student on a midwifery course is usually now new to examinations, but the format may differ from anything she was previously used to. The examination requires the student to demonstrate competence and sound clinical judgement, so preparation for it should not be rushed. The student may find it beneficial to draw up a plan of action to discuss with the course tutor. Students who have been away from formal study for a longer period may need more guidance.

Mental preparation
In our past experience early preparation for examination appears to be the most difficult to achieve except with a few individuals who have stringent self-discipline. Most students on

a new course find the first few weeks bewildering; they may be in a state of disorientation which continues for several months as they are faced with new challenges and tasks. This state of disorientation is very prevalent among midwifery students as the vast majority come to midwifery having held very responsible positions; returning to learner status takes a lot of adjustment. They may feel bereft of old familiar patterns and may experience feelings of uncertainty in their new role. But the student must quickly throw off these feelings and begin to think positively. The following statements may be useful to recall whenever she feels uncertain about her ability to complete the course.

> I have made a conscious decision to do this course therefore I am well motivated.

> I am currently experiencing some difficulty, but I can succeed; if there had been any doubts about my ability I would not have been selected.

> My level of knowledge may currently feel deficient but I cannot expect to learn all I need to know in such a short space of time or else there would be no need for me to do the course.

> I am perfectly capable of completing the course and passing the final examination as over 90 per cent of all students pass at the first attempt.

> All that I must do is work and apply myself to the course, putting theory into practice to become a competent practioner.

At the beginning of the course tutors try to instil into their students that it is better to study consistently throughout the course than to try to learn everything at once. Many research studies on learning and retention have shown that short periods of study, repetition, and a process of building on existing knowledge results in more information being retained. The following suggestions are intended as guidelines from which a personal programme can be built.

Guidelines

Try multiple short periods of study, each period not exceding forty minutes followed by a break of ten to fifteen minutes. Shorter periods fail to allow the brain sufficient time to absorb and organize material, while longer periods result in loss of detail.

At the end of the study period the student should test herself on aspects of the topic she has been studying. Testing and reviewing is an integral part of retention and reduces the quantity of information lost.

In a busy work schedule with shift patterns, social and domestic commitments it is not easy to allot time for study but setting aside time is *vital*. The student might begin by organizing a timetable with regular intervals of study that realistically assess what can be achieved on a daily or weekly basis. One of the most useful times is following a study day. After adequate rest and recreation the student should review her notes taken during the day, taking the opportunity to supplement these and reflect upon the day's proceedings.

After an adequate break the revised notes should be reread and summarized in brief note form to test recall and ensure that learning outcomes have been achieved. This pattern of events should be repeated two or three times to enable as much information as possible to be committed to memory. If this reflective process is repeated regularly, after some time the information will be easily recalled with only the occasional review.

To aid efficient review a system should be developed whereby brief notes are kept which may be filed under title heading with footnotes linking to other topics. If diagrams are used they should be simple enough to be easily reproduced and clearly labelled.

While notetaking is an important part of the learning exercise, the student must also be encouraged to read widely, particularly current publications. The information in these will be up to date and give current thoughts on established practice. This encourages students to think objectively and critically about their practice and develop skills necessary for discussion.

Becoming familiar with the examination format

Early introduction to the examination format is essential to enable the student to develop skills related to question answering, as she must satisfy the examiner of her ability to give adequate and professional care. She should be able to assess the needs of the patient and take appropriate action, safeguarding the wellbeing of mother, fetus and neonate in a competent and professional manner.

As part of the preparation for the qualifying examination most midwifery schools have regular tests, the format of the questions being the same as in the qualifying examination. When marking the papers the tutors take into consideration the student's experience, while also looking for accuracy of knowledge relevant to the amount of this experience. The grades allotted assist the student in identifying her areas of strengths and weaknesses. If she needs extra tuition she can negotiate with her tutor for remedial work as necessary.

Initially the questions may be answered with the aid of a textbook; but this prop should be used less and less until eventually the student is attempting questions under simulated examination conditions. These questions should be marked by a tutor and graded so that the student can see where progress is being made. At a later date the student may attempt the same questions in the light of further experience, and answer them in greater depth. In the long term the student will be able to select the most appropriate questions for her to answer and obtain maximum marks.

HANDWRITING, SPELLING AND PRESENTATION

This is covered in more detail in the next chapter, but worthy of a brief mention here. The student should try to develop a legible style of writing and organize her answers in a logical fashion. Examiners marking papers are always impressed with presentation as well as content.

OTHER AIDS TO LEARNING

Students must remember that books are not the only source of information, and effective use can be made of other aids. Tape/slides, films and video greatly enhance the learning process and can help absorb information.

Learning can be more fun with a friend. A contract could be set up between two partners whereby each has a commitment to research a given topic. A prearranged time could be made to meet and discuss the topic and exchange ideas.

The tutor as a resource tool can assist in learning. She is there for the student's benefit, so do not be afraid to make use of her knowledge. She can be a source of information to clarify specific points and may also help direct studies

The student should have adequate rest and some social activity: remember minds that are cluttered and preoccupied with problems and anxieties cannot be open and receptive to learning. If the student is well organized with a planned timetable and has set realistic goals for revision there will be time for socializing.

As the course nears the end and the examination day approaches the student must think about how and where to commence her revision programme. By now each student is aware of her own capabilities and therefore how much work is still left to be done; with a vast amount an early start to revision is needed. The student must decide on the number of hours each week she can give to revision.

As a guide to the final countdown start about twelve to sixteen weeks prior to the final examination. Within this time framework the student should aim to have completed revision two weeks before the examination day which would allow time for reflection and recap of specific areas.

The physical environment for studying is very individual, but it should be comfortable, with adequate lighting, warm but well ventilated, and with minimal distractions. It is best to sit at a desk or table to avoid fatigue and the temptation to fall asleep. If a full day is put aside for revision, there should be a limit of no more than six hours' study.

Finally, the student should reward herself for achieving her study goal – by doing something exciting and completely different.

Further reading

Ashman, S. and George, A. (1982). *Study and Learning: A Self-help Guide for Students*. Heinemann, London.

Buzan, T. (1982). *Use Your Head*. BBC Publications, London.

Cassie, W. and Constantine, T. (1972). *Students' Guide to Success*. Macmillan, London.

Freeman, R. (1982). *Mastering Study Skills*. Macmillan, London.

Maddox, H. (1967). *How to Study*. Pan Books, London.

Parsons, C. (1976). *How to Study Effectively*. Arrow Books, London.

Rowntree, D. (1976). *Learn How to Study*. Macdonald, London.

Chapter 3
General principles of examination technique

TYPES OF QUESTION

The types of question used in the midwifery qualifying examination are supply items, in that the student is being asked to supply information of her own rather than select information already given (as in multiple choice questions). They are confined to essay and short-answer questions.

The advantage of these types of questions is that the student's recall of information is tested and her ability to express ideas or show original thought can be assessed. It has also been shown that studying for these types of questions ensures that the subject matter is retained for longer periods.

It may be said that this is a subjective style of examination, but as all examiners attend an examiners' workshop before being appointed, and as a moderating committee has been set up to scrutinize any paper causing concern, this disadvantage is minimized.

Essay questions (see chapter 8) can ask for comparisons, decisions, explanations, causes, effects or relationships and discussions. They may be extended, usually one question covering all the marks given or restricted, that is, divided into specific parts each with its own weighting.

Short-answer questions (see chapter 8) are used to assess powers of recall. They can ask for a direct answer, a short explanation or a list.

General principles of examination technique

Whatever the type of question asked, provided it is read carefully to avoid misinterpretation, the student having had enough practice during her training period, should be able to elicit what precisely the question is asking for.

PAPER AND QUESTION PLANNING

Before planning an individual question, the student must first decide which questions from the examination paper she plans to answer. Selection of the most appropriate questions to be answered is of paramount importance.

Before reading the questions, look for any specific instructions regarding the paper as a whole. How many questions must be answered? How many questions from each section? How long should be spent on each?

Read the paper carefully
On first reading the paper, form no opinions and write nothing. On the second reading, underline what you consider to be the key words in each question. Consider the type of question being asked. Is it an extended-response question which asks you to discuss or express your opinions? These questions are not usually weighted. You may feel that although you would be happy to participate in a verbal discussion you would not be able to demonstrate your knowledge so well in writing in a broad-topic question. Should this be the case you my feel more at ease with the restricted-response question where each of the parts indicates the percentage of marks allocated to it. Finally, read the paper through once more marking your selection of questions to be answered.

Individual questions
You are now in a position to commence planning individual questions. There are two ways to approach this: plan all the questions selected before commencing to write the paper; or plan the first question, write it, then follow by planning the

next question, write it, and continue in this manner until the paper is completed. Either way is acceptable, provided that *you have followed this plan before and it has worked for you*. The qualifying examination is *not* the time to start experimenting.

Plan a short introduction to the question stating where you are going and how you are going to get there. Plan the body of the question by following the introduction, and the conclusion to reiterate the main points raised. Check whether any weighting of the question had been taken into consideration. Is there too much information for a part that carries 20 per cent of the marks, and only a small amount for the part that carries 80 per cent? Check that where it says list, items *are* listed; if it says discuss, have opposing viewpoints been expressed; where it asks for an opinion, has it been given? Is the argument written logically, and opinions backed up with solid fact? Has the question been answered in a logical sequence, or are all the facts jumbled together? An answer that flows from one point to another in an ordered way shows clarity of thought and good question planning, and therefore creates a favourable impression.

Finally, the question should be reread once more to determine whether it has in fact been answered, or whether you only think you have. It is all too easy in the stress of the moment to misinterpret the question or to go off at a tangent. Having decided that the question plan does answer the question, proceed to the next question plan.

QUESTION CONSTRUCTION

Spelling

Spelling errors, while not proving that one is incapable of safe practice, nevertheless create a bad impression. It is important therefore to pay attention to this aspect of your work.

If there are certain words that you consistently spell incorrectly, it is a good idea to compile a notebook of such

General principles of examination technique

words during training and review them on a daily basis, so that with continual repetition their correct spelling will be learnt.

Careless spelling is, however, a separate issue, and one very good reason for reading the examination paper through carefully on completion to correct any misspelt words.

Punctuation

Use punctuation marks where appropriate, punctuating long sentences carefully to make the meaning clear.

Grammar

One either knows one's grammar or one does not. If this has proved a problem in the past, the use of a grammar book or undertaking a suitable course should help.

One common error is to switch tenses one or more times during the course of a question. Practise at question or essay writing should help with this problem, and again reading the paper through on completion allows for correction where required.

Headings

The use of headings is a personal preference. If you feel that they aid presentation and logicality of thought, provided they are relevant and do not interrupt the flow, they are perfectly permissible. Headings are possibly of more relevance in the restricted-answer questions to introduce each section, rather than in the extended question where an essay-style reply is more usual. Headings may also be useful in the short-answer questions to aid in the presentation of short, precise facts.

If headings are used, they should be short and underlined using either the same colour ink or a contrasting colour.

Underlining

Other than underlining headings it is occasionally useful to stress a word or phrase to emphasize a point. Do not, however, underline so frequently that it interrupts the flow of the answer, or spoils the presentation.

Sentences

When writing a paper, it is a good idea to keep sentences short and snappy. Reading a long involved sentence, especially one that is poorly punctuated, can obscure a valid point and leave the examiner somewhat confused and frustrated, not to say breathless! Generally speaking, the shorter the sentence, the clearer the meaning. But this concept should not be confused with a note style of presentation.

Paragraphs

A paragraph should be used to cover one aspect of the topic under consideration. A new aspect starts a new paragraph, usually with a new line, indenting the sentence approximately one inch from the margin. Paragraphs are particularly important in the extended essay question where headings may not be appropriate.

Quotations and referencing

If an author is quoted, the quotation must be accurate and place in inverted commas. If the exact words cannot be remembered do not quote, but if the student is sure of the theme of an author this could be used in place of quotation as follows:

> O'Driscoll is very much in favour of augmentation of labour to facilitate delivery within his stated optimum time.

This should be followed by the initial and the surname of the author, the name of the book and the year of publication if known. Material used from an article would be referenced in the same way.

Abbreviations

Abbreviations are acceptable, but the correct formula must be adhered to.

> The abbreviation must be in common use, for example, PPH.

General principles of examination technique 17

The first time the phrase is used it should be written in full with the abbreviation in brackets immediately after, for example, postpartum haemorrhage (PPH).

Slang expressions in common use that abbreviate a word should never be used, for example, 'flat baby'.

CONTENT

Obviously the content will change depending on the question, but several factors will be appropriate to each one. Where relevant:

State the facts.
Apply the rules.
Apply the Code of Practice.
Apply the Code of Professional Conduct.
If a judgement is called for – make it.
If an opinion is asked for – give it.
Illustrate a fact with personal experience.
Quote statistics where appropriate.
Quote research where appropriate.
Use diagrams if appropriate.
Avoid irrelevant information.

In this way the answer should cover all the major areas that show knowledge of the subject, together with attitude and ability to make decisions.

Finally, if any controversial material is used, state the facts clearly to ensure that the examiner knows that this is controversial. It may also be appropriate to give your opinion on such material if it can be backed up with facts or experience.

DIAGRAMS

Use of diagrams can illustrate a point or a number of points being made and, used judiciously, can also save time. Any diagram used should be drawn in proportion, be fully labelled and be an accurate representation of the part being illustrated.

Diagrams need not be works of art: a simple outline will suffice, and in all likelihood be just as clear, if not clearer.

Graphs to show statistics are also diagrams and can be used most effectively to illustrate certain types of questions.

The most important point to remember is that it takes practice to be able to reproduce any diagram accurately at will.

When using a diagram let it speak for itself, for example describing the anatomy of the pelvic floor. If a full and *accurate* diagram is used less words will be required in the explanation.

TIMING

The timing of the paper is crucial. A candidate who does not complete a paper is in danger of failing the examination, although this is not always so.

Reading the question paper through as described on page 13 will take approximately five minutes. Allow approximately five to six minutes to plan each major question, and approximately two minutes for each short-answer question. Allow approximately seven to ten minutes to read through the paper on completion and correct any obvious errors.

The total planning/revision time is thus approximately forty minutes. The total time available to write the paper is thus approximately 140 minutes. This allows thirty-six to thirty-eight minutes for each major question, and approximately seven to eight minutes for each short-answer question.

This does not seem very long, especially for the major questions. However, if you have planned thoroughly, there will be no prolonged pauses while you consider what to write next, wish you had written it in a different order, or even tried

General principles of examination technique

another question entirely. It should also reduce careles errors because one is working in an organized manner, to an organized plan.

Timing only comes with practice, which is one of the reasons for intra-course examinations and tests.

Concentration levels can also affect timing, being higher at the beginning of an examination and possibly just before the end. It is worth considering, therefore, answering the questions that possibly pose the greatest difficulty at the beginning and leaving the short-answer questions, which are concise and to the point, until the end.

Slow writers may have more difficulty in completing the paper on time, as may students who have a more 'wordy' style of writing. It is of the *utmost importance* that problems such as these are highlighted early on in the course and steps taken to rectify them.

HANDWRITING

Handwriting is important, and though no one style should be preferred, legibility and neatness create a favourable first impression. Consider that any one examiner may be marking twenty answer books, which amounts to sixty main questions and twenty short-answer questions. This is a considerable task, and although content must be more important than clarity of handwriting, the latter assists the examiner to concentrate on the subject matter being presented, rather than struggling to decipher each word.

Remember, if the examiners cannot read a student's handwriting, they cannot assess her level of knowledge and expertise. This will not disadvantage them, only you.

FINAL SHOPPING DAY BEFORE THE EXAMINATION

Check that you have all the equipment you will need to take into the examination room.

> Pens
> Pencils
> Pencil sharpener
> Rubber
> Alternative colour pen
> Ruler
> White paint (e.g. 'Tipp Ex')
> Coloured pencils or crayons for diagrams.
> Sweets (if it is felt these will aid concentration)
> A carton of juice with a straw

Any of the above-mentioned items that are not in the student's possession at this time should be purchased well in advance to save panic the night before the examination when shops are shut.

THE DAY BEFORE THE EXAMINATION

Collect together all the items needed for the following day (see above). Use some kind of container, even a plastic bag, to put all the items into. Check that you have your entrance card to hand, giving your candidate's number and the venue of the examination.

Ensure that you know the best route to the examination venue and the time you are required to present yourself. Calculate the time it will take you to get there, allowing for factors such as rush hour, the vagaries of the public transport system, or the time it will take you to find a parking space or change a wheel on a car. Plan to arrive at the examination centre at least thirty minutes before you have to; you can always go for a cup of coffee to pass the extra time.

If you live a long way from the centre, it may be worth

General principles of examination technique

considering staying with a colleague who is closer, especially if the weather is severe. Having to leave home at 5 am and still arriving at the examination centre thirty minutes late has happened to more than one candidate when there were snowdrifts to overcome.

Have sufficient money available for any fares or emergencies that may arise, and extra to join colleagues for a coffee or a drink after the examination to help unwind.

ON ENTERING THE EXAMINATION ROOM

This is the moment of truth. During the next few hours you will be called upon to demonstrate the knowledge and understanding you have worked so hard to achieve over your training period.

Your mouth may feel dry, you may feel sick, your mind may feel blank. DON'T PANIC. Remember, everyone is on the same side. The examination papers have not been designed to trap you or to find out what you *don't* know, rather the reverse it is important to establish what you do know so that an assessment may be made as to whether you will be safe to practise as a midwife.

If you have applied yourself to your studies during the preceding months, you will have gained ample knowledge to answer the questions. Take a few deep breaths, perhaps employ a method of relaxation, to calm the mind and relax the body.

Whether or not specifically instructed to do so, rule margins in your answer book and enter your candidate number on each page. Write on each side of the paper and always use a new page when starting a new question.

Finally, GOOD LUCK!

Chapter 4
The viva voce

Gone are the days when the candidate was 'grilled' by two examiners, one of whom was originally an obstetrician, the other a midwife teacher. As both examiners were responsible for marking the candidate's two examination papers, part of the twenty-minute session was often used to clarify or enlarge upon some aspect of the written paper.

Since the change in format in 1986, the viva is conducted completely separately from the written examination, with one midwife teacher who has no knowledge of the student's results or ability. Its main purpose is to assess aspects of midwifery that cannot be included in the written paper; 100 marks are allocated to it.

The viva takes the form of a discussion and gives the examiner the opportunity to explore, with the candidate, wider issues in midwifery that may be difficult to determine in a written paper. It attempts to assess four aspects of the candidate's ability:

> decision-making
> judgement,
> communication, and
> attitude.

Decision-making and judgement, which seem to be almost synonymous, test one's ability to think critically, anticipate

The viva voce

difficulties and solve problems. The ability to communicate is important to the midwife and she must be able to show that she can impart knowledge. During the viva, after an initial period of nervousness, the candidate will usually have relaxed sufficiently to settle into conversation, demonstrating knowledge and communicating thoughts and ideas.

The final aspect being assessed is attitude. This can be attitude to:

the woman and the care she receives,
the responsibilities of the midwife to the profession,
the midwife's role as educator, and
how the midwife might influence change.

Twenty minutes gives ample time to explore these aspects, and is generally found to be quite enjoyable and often exhilarating to both candidate and examiner. As a two-way process, much can be gained by both contributors. Marked out of 100, a mark of fifty or above indicates that the candidate has shown the required level of ability.

Another useful innovation is that the names of the examiners are displayed on a table plan. This allows the candidate to know in advance the examiner's name, making the occasion more personal.

THE EXAMINER

The examiner, no longer anonymous, has two main responsibilites. First, she must show fairness to the candidate, and give her the opportunity in an artificial situation, and under some degree of stress and anxiety, to relate the information asked for. Second, the examiner has a responsibility to the midwifery profession and the future of midwifery.

Aspects of research and the influence it has on practice are important issues, and the ability to relate some knowledge of these is important. The examiner often gains useful information, and can use the time as an opportunity to broaden her own knowledge by learning about local practice, and thereby educating herself.

OVERCOMING NERVES

No matter how many times the student is reassured that the viva will be 'OK', and in most cases enjoyed, it would not be normal if she were not slightly anxious. In some ways the viva resembles an interview, and as such is accompanied by a certain degree of nervousness. The candidate wants to do her best, and needs to be able to concentrate. She should choose an outfit that is comfortable, tidy, and reasonably smart. If she looks good she will feel confident and concentrate better on the viva. Under stress we sometimes gesticulate and wave our hands about, often without being aware of our actions. If that seems to be a problem, the student should try gently clasping her hands together and resting them on her lap, or sit on them! For a dry mouth, suck a mint or even chew some gum *before* going in to the examiner.

TRIAL RUNS

Students often feel that they have had insufficient practice at vivas. Certainly it helps to have a few trial runs to get an idea of what it is like, and it may be helpful to role-play the viva situation with colleagues. What is most important is to gain confidence in speaking and talking to other people. Trial runs often help, although in reality one is not fully prepared as one does not know what the examiner will ask. Vivas, like interviews, are all different, but each situation may challenge the student's ability to recall facts, recount incidences, show an ability to make decisions, and test knowledge and attitude. No learning situation need be wasted, but remember, time spent being educated and 'trained' as a midwife is for the years ahead, to encourage critical thinking and safe practice – and within a twenty-minute session some of that will emerge.

All that remains is to make up one's mind to enjoy the viva. Remember, it could be the examiner's first time too, and she may be more nervous than the student!

Chapter 5
Weighting, marking and moderating

PROFILE OF THE EXAMINERS

As already stated in this book, the examiners are practising, experienced midwifery teachers, who have attended an 'art of examiners' course for marking examination papers. Their main interest is in ensuring that the standards and safe practices of midwifery are maintained. There is no limit to how many candidates are allowed to attain the standard, therefore provided a student's answers are relevant to the question asked, and contain adequate and accurate information, she should be successful.

WEIGHTING

Each of the two papers are marked out of 400 marks, 200 or above indicating that the candidate has reached the correct level of ability for each paper. As stated clearly in the instructions to candidates, three of the five long questions should be attempted and four of the eight short questions.

Each long question is worth 100 marks, that is a quarter of the total marks available, so the candidate should allocate a quarter of the examination time to each of the long answers, approximately forty-five minutes. This time should include planning of the answer, presentation and checking through afterwards.

A proportion of the long questions are known as *restricted-*

Weighting, marking and moderating

response questions, and have the total 100 marks subdivided, allocating a percentage of the marks to different aspects of the question. This is very useful for the candidates as they are then aware how much each part of the question is worth and therefore how much of the forty-five minutes should be allocated to each specific part.

The remaining long questions are not divided into parts and are known as *extended-response questions* (in other words 100 per cent questions). These tend to be discussion questions, so it is more difficult to assess which areas of the subject are to be expanded upon. The articulate student who enjoys discussion, and tends not to digress, is best suited to answer these questions.

Since the new examination came into being in July 1986, statistics indicate that the long questions that are subdivided into parts are more popular than the long questions with no subdivision.

Short-answer questions, each worth twenty-five marks are the final questions on the paper. Each answer should take approximately ten minutes. The fact that each answer is worth twenty-five marks, clearly indicates that they should be relatively short, covering approximately a half to one side of paper depending on the size of the writing. Answers should contain the vital points, without digression, especially if the topic is related to a midwifery emergency.

Clearly the weighting of the questions can be used for the benefit of the candidates and their examination technique. It is vital that the appropriate time is allocated to each answer so that other answers are not jeopardized by having insufficient time to finish all the questions, thereby inevitably not only losing but throwing away marks. Students are well advised to practise examination questions with special attention to the time taken for their answers.

THE VIVA

This is covered more fully in Chapter 4.

MARKING

Each examiner has ten to fifteen papers to mark, either paper 1 or paper 2. Before marking the papers the examiner will draw up an answer plan for each question to contain the most important points that must be included in the answer to the question. This is especially important when it is a life-threatening situation, such as postpartum haemorrhage or cord prolapse. The answer plan will also contain less essential points, but nevertheless relevant to the question. The examiner will then read the candidate's answer and allocate marks accordingly. The examiner's answer plan will be based on her own knowledge of the topic, plus research that she will have carried out to supplement and update her own knowledge and experience as appropriate.

It cannot be overstressed that *marks will not be given for information that is irrelevant to the question*. Therefore it is extremely important for candidates to ensure that their answer is relevant, otherwise they are wasting valuable time during their examination. It is essential to read the question carefully before planning the answer.

As the examiner is marking ten to fifteen papers, with four questions on each paper, it is a good examination technique to ensure that writing is legible, and important points are highlighted by underlining them, thus giving them more emphasis (see also Chapter 3). It is also helpful if candidates read the instructions carefully.

Examiners marking *national papers* tend to mark all the same numbered questions at one time rather than a candidate's entire paper. That is to say, if an examiner marks question 1 of the first paper she will then mark all the other answers to question 1. This will give her an overall standard of the candidates response to

Weighting, marking and moderating

that question. After she has marked each question, she will allocate marks out of 100, *fifty being the mark required to attain a satisfactory standard for each question*. The maximum marks for a complete paper total 400, *the necessary standard being 200*. It is, therefore, possible to do badly in one question, but still attain a satisfactory overall standard.

MODERATING

To ensure that each candidate is given a fair chance of being successful in the examination, a moderating committee meet after each examination has been marked but prior to any results being distributed.

Papers sent for moderation fall into one of the following two categories:

when a candidate's paper is awarded less than 210 marks;
any paper about which the examiner has doubts.

The moderating committee, which meets at the English National Board, comprises seven to eight of the examiners who have been involved in marking the current papers. They are from all regions of the country to eliminate any geographical bias towards midwifery/obstetric practice.

The committee can receive any number of papers from each examiner, but in reality this tends to be two to three from each. The moderators work in pairs and look at the papers that have been sent to them, discussing specific areas of concern. Following discussion, a decision is made on whether a satisfactory standard has been attained but if they cannot reach agreement, the paper is put to the whole committee to decide on its outcome. Within the moderating committee, members will not moderate any papers they themselves have originally marked.

The examination is not designed to 'trick' candidates into failing. If the candidate has a good examination technique, such as proper timing (even being ruthless and cutting short a favourite topic), sticking to the point when answering questions, constantly referring back to the question, looking at key words such as 'discuss', 'list', 'describe', and ensuring that the answer given is relevant, the examiner will be awarding the candidate marks, therefore the chances are that she will attain the necessary standard in the examination.

Chapter 6

Midwifery qualifying examination: Differences in the examination system

ENGLAND

There have been considerable changes in the last few years to the format of the examination papers. The current papers have a more standardized format than either that of Scotland or Northern Ireland.

The purpose of the midwifery qualifying examination is to assess the candidate's ability as a midwife to work both on her own and as a member of a team – in other words as a competent practitioner.

The present system, introduced in July 1986, is for an interim period while a more radical review of the educational process in midwifery is pursued within the Board's policy framework. The arrangement of the midwifery qualifying examination must be in line with current midwifery practice and encourage the candidates to express opinion and ideas.

The examination consists of two written papers, each of three hours' duration and an oral examination (viva voce) of twenty minutes.

Three out of five long questions should be answered regardless of whether they are restricted- or extended-response questions. The sixth question contains eight topics, four of which should be answered taking approximately ten minutes over each.

The two written papers are designed to sample the full range of theoretical teaching and clinical individualized experience. This includes the concepts of planned continuity of care, and care for the mother and baby as a single unit.

The variety of question type, restricted response with in-question weighting, extended response and short topic questions provide the candidate with a good opportunity to show her range and grasp of the subject. The viva voce provides a rare opportunity as a forum for discussion.

SCOTLAND

General education in Scotland is somewhat different from that in England. Following O level, a higher grade examination is taken in the next year and is less specialized than the English A level examination. Similarly, Scottish universities offer a more general degree course – often composed of up to nine modules, only some of which are carried forward from year to year.

Nursing and midwifery education tends to follow this philosophy of a broad rather than a very specialized approach according to their statutory body, the National Board for Nursing, Midwifery and Health Visiting for Scotland (Kirkmanm, 1986, personal communication). Some of the examination papers do, however, demand very specific responses.

The two papers for the midwifery qualifying examination follow the modern ideal of individualized patient/family-centred care. Several questions often relate to a brief case history of social as well as obstetric details, which is given at the beginning of the paper. Paper 1 is broadly concerned with midwifery, obstetric abnormalities, labour with applied anatomy and physiology, although there are quite wide variations as can be seen in the examples given in Chapter 8. Paper 2 sets out to test the candidate's knowledge of: paediatrics, social services and education in both community health and parentcraft.

Both papers usually contain four compulsory questions, each

Midwifery qualifying examination

carrying twenty-five marks. Occasionally there are five questions, each carrying twenty marks. The individual structure may also widely vary from question to question – some may carry twenty-five marks as a whole, while others may be subdivided into various parts, each with its own weighting.

The examination may also reflect the two major differences between Scottish and English training practices: the community placement is of four weeks duration; and clinical teachers may be mentioned in the papers.

Each examiner receives a sheet of key facts accompanying the paper to be marked. This contains the essential facts which should appear in the answer and is an attempt to achieve a more standardized marking system from the examiners. The system is not so rigid as it may first appear as key facts are not all inclusive and credit should be given for other relevant facts in an answer.

NORTHERN IRELAND

The National Board for Nursing, Midwifery and Health Visiting also sets two papers as the final examination for admission to Part 10 of the Register – Midwifery.

The first paper contains eight compulsory questions, each carrying twenty-five marks, some of which may be subdivided for weighting. This paper asks for factual information and a description of applied anatomy and physiology. Prenatal, natal and postnatal and paediatric subjects are covered.

The second paper is longer and concentrates on the role of the midwife in both normal and abnormal situations that can arise. Section A of this paper is compulsory and carries 100 marks. Four questions make up Section B, especially related to the midwife's role in normal and emergency care, three of these must be attempted. The third part, Section C, has two questions, one of which must be answered. A paediatric question is always included, but the second may be related to any aspect of midwifery. Again each question can be subdivided and weighted in varying ways. Examples are given in Chapter 8.

Chapter 7
Advanced Diploma of Midwifery Examination

The Advanced Diploma of Midwifery (ADM) was introduced in 1971 by the Central Midwives Board, now extinct. However, the course objectives were not clearly defined and the course content may have been ambiguous. The qualification was considered to be of a lower standard than the professional part of the Midwife Tutors Diploma. Some members of the profession saw it as the acceptable qualification for promotion in the clinical and the administration fields, whilst others considered it was the preparation for the Midwife Tutors Diploma (MTD).

In addition to these areas of concern within the profession itself, the sectors of further and higher education did not accept this certificate as an entry qualification into academic courses. The ADM was then subjected to a major revision in 1980, following the recommendations of the Education Committee of the Royal College of Midwives. The main objective of the Diploma now is to prepare the midwife to enter a multidisciplinary teaching course such as the Postgraduate Certificate in Adult Education.

The curriculum embraces the following modules: midwifery and paediatrics, and behavioural sciences.

MIDWIFERY AND PAEDIATRICS

The Central Midwives Board's Directives (October 1980) state that in preparation for the examination the theory and practice should be studied in detail consistent with the fact that a minimum of two years' clinical experience must precede the Diploma, and that must be recently obtained. All relevant aspects of these essential subjects as well as a knowledge of research, should be related to developments in practice. The student should have a working knowledge in those areas of biological sciences relating to the curriculum. This section of the course should constitute half the curriculum time, and should cover related anatomy and physiology, embryology, fetal development, together with neonatal physiology and changes at birth. The application of microbiology and immunology should also be included.

BEHAVIOURAL SCIENCES

The study of these areas should facilitate the student's understanding of the psychology, sociology and social policy relevant to their responsibilities as experienced midwives. This necessitates being informed about family units, their cultural and social environments, as well as being aware of the current health and social policies.

THE MIDWIFERY PROFESSION

Students should become familiar with the historical background of the development of their profession, seeing how legislation controls practice, and being aware of how midwifery education has developed alongside and interrelated with the growth of other health professions.

Other changes were made to achieve academic credibility. As well as lengthening the course and including the behavioural sciences, teaching methods appropriate to the development of independent and critical thinking are currently used.

The award of the ADM involves the assessment of four in-course assignments, two of which are presented for the final discussion after the written examination as well as the final examination itself. The purpose of these assessments are to ensure that the relationship between the needs of society and the quality of service provided by the profession continues to be of the highest possible standard.

Chapter 8
Sample questions and answers

INTRODUCTION

In this chapter no attempt has been made to answer the selected questions fully, but rather to give the student guidelines on what important facts she should be attempting to highlight before setting pen to paper. Much more emphasis has been placed on answering full-length questions as these usually present the biggest problem to the student. Where appropriate an outline of essential information has been included to give some idea of what the examiner could reasonably expect to find in the answer. Where a diagram will help to illustrate the answer, or provide a complete answer, it has been included in the answer plan.

To make full use of this book, the student should study some of the answer plans then answer some questions without referring to the guidelines. She can then check the information in the answer plan to ensure that all the essential material has been included.

Short questions often present less problems, although there is no time to include non-essential information. The topics are simply listed and candidates are requested to write on four out of eight topics, for example:

(a) lochia;
(b) Entonox;

(c) policies for the identification of babies in hospital;
(d) use of blood transfusion for a childbearing mother;
(e) sore nipples;
(f) consumption of alcohol in pregnancy;
(g) ophthalmia neonatorum.

(from the English National Board, January 1988 paper)

In a different situation some of these topics could constitute a complete long answer and it is left to the student to pick those aspects she feels should be included. The examples given are only a guide. Where an answer should include definite information this has been indicated. If the topic refers to an emergency situation, such as antepartum haemorrhage, postpartum haemorrhage, eclampsia, etc., a definition of the condition would be expected with an outline of the emergency management undertaken by the midwife to maintain safety.

It is recommended that approximately ten minutes is devoted to each short question. Practising these will ensure that the student is more easily able to get the timing right.

Appendix 1 gives all the exam papers set by the three National Boards (England, Scotland, Northern Ireland) since the examination format was changed in 1986, without answer plans. The student should try answering some of these to gain practice, being careful to time her answers, as forty-five minutes is all that is allowed in the real examination to answer one complete long question. Having completed the answer the student should either check the information herself, ask her tutor to check some for her, or ask a colleague to help. Another useful ploy is to do an answer plan only, looking at what information should be included. These answer plans are also useful for revision purposes.

Unless otherwise stated all the questions used in this section have been taken from previous English National Board examination papers (dates and marks are given for reference) and published in their entirety.

Sample questions and answers

LONG QUESTIONS

Q.1 (a) **List the aims of antenatal care.** (10)
(b) **Describe in detail how a midwife may achieve these aims.** (90)

(*ENB, 4.11.86*)   100

A. This is a fairly popular question and should present no problems to the student provided that she answers the question. From the weighting of the question the student can see that the majority of time available should be allocated to *part (b)* that is 90 per cent of the available forty-five minutes. A plan of action is essential for this kind of question and enables the student to organize her thoughts into some semblance of order.

The important points to note in part (a) are that the student is asked to *list* the aims of antenatal care. An aim is a broad statement of intent signifying expected or desirable outcome, so the list should include the following:

(i) maintenance of health and wellbeing of mother and baby;
(ii) preparation of the mother and her partner for labour;
(iii) preparation of the mother for infant feeding;
(iv) preparation of both partners for their new role (or extended role) as parents.

Part (b) which earns the majority of the marks, should relate directly to the list of aims outlined and should bring out all aspects of the midwife's role in providing antenatal care. If each of the aims is made a separate heading, this can be used to expand the answer including all the duties the midwife performs with a full description of the way in which she achieves them, thereby bringing in the detail requested in the question.

Apart from detailing how the midwife's normal skills are utilized to maintain fetal and maternal wellbeing, consideration should be given to communication skills, continuity of care and liaison with other health personnel in achieving the aims.

Education of the mother and her partner plays a major role in antental care and the student must be careful to include this in her answer.

Q.2 Describe the role of the midwife in achieving the aims of antenatal care. (100)

(ENB, 16.3.87)

A. This is a very similar question to the one above but with a 100 per cent weighting. It would be very easy in this question not to be organized and not to answer the question properly. As the question is concerned with the role of the midwife in achieving the aims of antenatal care some definition of these aims should be given. As in the previous question, a list of aims would be appropriate allowing the student to expand the list as before.

It may be relevant here to reiterate that the midwife's role includes all aspects of the normal care that she would give to any pregnant woman. Questions which include the 'role of the midwife' often seem to put the student into an immediate panic situation, but if thought out logically are very straightforward to answer. One word of warning: do not neglect the role of the midwife in identifying high risk or abnormal conditions and referring them to the appropriate person. Also, look a little wider than the normal antenatal clinic visits and include such aspects as suitable place for confinement, follow-up non-clinic attendants, the midwife's role as educator, utilization of other team members, antenatal preparation for parenthood and promotion of breast-feeding as listed in the aims.

Q.3 Discuss the significance of blood tests that may be carried out during pregnancy. (100)

(ENB, 8.9.86)

A. This question demands that consideration be given to all blood tests that may be carried out in pregnancy from the time of booking to delivery. It may be easy just to concentrate only

Sample questions and answers

on the blood tests performed at the booking visit, but the student must be careful to look beyond this.

A useful strategy for the student would be to make a rough list of all the blood tests that she knows may be performed, then select those that are carried out regularly and devise a system of priority. Routine tests should be covered first, less common ones being dealt with subsequently, for example:

(i) *Routine blood tests:*
   booking bloods (see following answer);
   subsequent routine tests (see following answer).
(ii) *Other blood tests*
   serum uric acid;
   human placental lactogen;
   oestriols;
   platelets, etc.

In the answer it is important to state which blood test is being considered, at what stage of pregnancy it may be performed, the reason for it being done, and the *significance* of undertaking the test (in other words, what would it indicate if the result were abnormal?). For common tests such as haemoglobin estimation it would be reasonable to expect the student to know the normal values and how to document them accurately.

Other considerations should be given as to whether all the tests performed are really necessary, and the ethics and implications of carrying out any blood test without the consent of the person concerned. This is particularly topical at the moment with the suggestion that all pregnant women should be screened for the HIV/AIDS virus. The student should be particularly aware of the significance of this to the woman, her unborn baby, other members of her family and her midwifery attendants.

Important points in answering this question are to get the balance of information right and constantly to refer to the significance of undertaking the particular blood test you may be discussing, bringing out both good and contentious points, and not digressing from the question asked.

Q.4 Discuss the importance of routine blood tests in the antenatal period. (100)

(Adapted from ENB paper)

A. A number of blood tests are taken during the antenatal period, but here the student should note that she is only required to talk about *routine* tests. These include the following:

(i) *Booking bloods*
ABO group;
haemoglobin;
rhesus and atypical antibodies;
serology for syphilis (TPHA, VDRL, etc.);
rubella antibody titre;
electrophoresis for haemoglobinopathies.

Detection of HIV antibodies may also be considered routine in some units.

(ii) *Subsequent routine blood tests*
alphafetoprotein (may be carried out on the booking visit in some units);
repeat haemoglobin;
repeat rhesus antibodies.

Each of these blood tests and their significance needs to be described. Other blood tests which may be routine in the student's own unit should also be included, for example, blood sugar estimation, human placental lactogen, oestrogens, although the student should be prepared to argue her case for considering these to be routine.

The discussion should include the adverse effects on either mother, or fetus, or other adverse effects to which lack of diagnosis may lead and benefits that may result from them being done, for example, if a woman who is known to be rhesus negative does not have her blood tested for rhesus antibodies at regular intervals she could be developing antibodies that may adversely effect her fetus. Treatment would not be instituted, and in severe cases intrauterine or early neonatal death might

Sample questions and answers

ensue. For the want of a simple, routine test the effect on the family could be devastating. The positive side to detecting rhesus antibodies is that extra monitoring and treatment can be instigated and reduce the problems for the fetus.

Included in the answer should be a discussion of the practical and ethical issues involved in performing some of these tests, such as informed consent for tests like alphafetoprotein and HIV, their cost-effectiveness, and the implications of a positive result on the family.

Q.5	(a) Outline the anatomy of the non-pregnant uterus.	(25)
	(b) Describe the changes in the uterus that occur during pregnancy.	(50)
	(c) Outline the changes that occur in the uterus during the ten days following delivery.	(25)
(*ENB, 8.9.86*)		100

A. The weighting of this question gives some indication as to the length of time that should be spent on each area. The first and third parts of the question ask only for an outline so they should be brief, while the second part of the question asks for a description, so the answer should have more detail.

Part (a) asks for an outline of the anatomy of *non-pregnant uterus*. Anatomy questions require the student to describe the organ both macroscopically and microscopically, its position and relationship to other organs, its function, and its blood, nerve and lymph supply. A diagram could be very useful here.

For part (b) the student must give consideration to factors that bring about major changes in the uterus during pregnancy, such as hypertrophy and hypoplasia, changes in the lining of the uterus, differentiation of muscle layers, hormonal influences, increased blood supply etc., contents of the uterus, reasons for these changes occurring and how they relate to the non-pregnant uterus (in size, shape, etc.).

Part (c) requires the student to outline the changes that occur

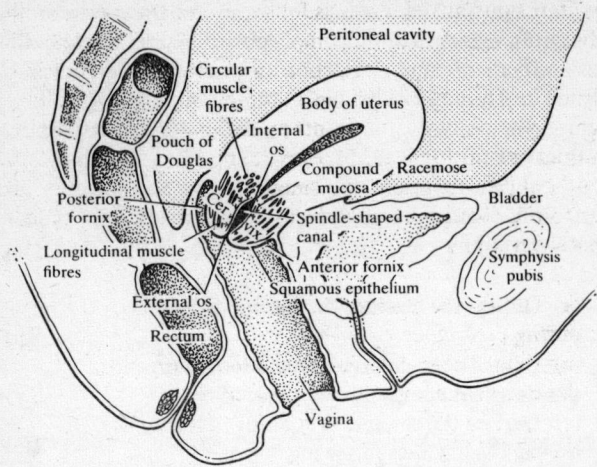

Fig. 1 Outline of anatomy of non-pregnant uterus

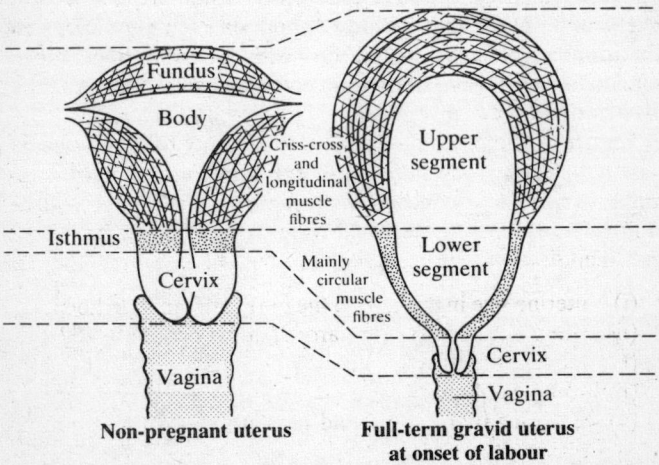

Fig. 2 Comparison of non-pregnant uterus and uterus at full-term (drawings not to scale)

in the uterus during the ten days following delivery. It would be beneficial to commence at completion of the third stage of labour and to include retraction, ischaemia, phagocytosis, autolysis, involution and lochia. Outline also how the midwife recognizes the normality of events by the rate of involution.

Throughout this answer the examiner will be looking at the student's ability to relate the anatomy of the non-pregnant uterus to the changes taking place in both pregnancy and the postnatal period.

Q.6 (a) **Outline the changes that occur in the uterus during pregnancy.** (40)
(b) **What factors influence variations in uterine size during the latter half of pregnancy?** (60)

(*ENB, 14.9.87*) 100

A. Part (a) may be answered in much the same way as part (b) of the previous question, except here the student is asked to *outline* for 40 per cent of the question, therefore no comparison needs to be made. It is fairly common for some physiology to be included in examination questions alongside the more practical application as this gives a good guide to the student's ability to inter-relate.

For part (b) the student needs to consider why the pregnant woman and her uterus are being examined and palpated and what it is hoped to find. An attempt is being made to confirm normality, or identify abnormality, and the following should be considered:

(i) uterine size in relation to the period of amenorrhoea;
(ii) size of fetus – growth retarded, growth accelerated?
(iii) number of fetuses;
(iv) volume of liquor;
(v) shape of uterus – lie and presentation, localization of placenta;
(vi) state of maternal health – this may indirectly influence fetal size.

The student should bring out how the above factors may influence uterine size remembering that she is considering only the *latter* half of pregnancy.

Q.7 (a) **What are the aims of parentcraft education in the antenatal period?** (20)
  (b) **Describe a programme to achieve these aims.** (50)
  (c) **What facilities should be available for antenatal parentcraft education within a health district?** (30)

(*ENB, 9.9.86*) 100

A. Part (a) gains only 20 per cent of the available marks, so does not require specific details. The aims should be listed (as below) with an explanatory sentence for each; this would take the nine or ten minutes allowed. Give information to cover all aspects of:

(i) antenatal care;
(ii) preparation for labour;
(iii) postnatal care;
(iv) preparation for parenthood;
(v) allaying fears.

Bring out the opportunity this gives to educate both parents in all aspects of care.

Part (b) requires a straightforward description of a programme to meet the above needs. Half the available time should be spent in answering this section.

It is important not to cite a programme from one's own hospital unless it meets the needs indicated in the first section. Obviously a programme that is known may fulfil all the needs, or could be used as a basis for an answer.

Included in this section should be some comment on how parentcraft classes would be conducted in relation to flexibility within them, discussions, and accommodation of any special needs of the groups as all groups are different.

Sample questions and answers

For part (c) it is important to note that the student is not asked for what facilities *are* available within a health district but what *should* be available. This gives her an opportunity to use her imagination a little and bring out her knowledge of what facilities are available as well of those she feels would be of benefit but are not generally available. Aspects covered could include:

(i) the different varieties of settings available;
(ii) different types of classes available, including facilities for those with 'special' needs (such as different ethnic groups, first-time parents, adoptive parents);
(iii) space and equipment;
(iv) staff;
(v) provision of crêches;
(vi) inclusion of voluntary groups, etc.

Q.8 Parentcraft education will need to differ according to various client groups. Discuss this statement.

100

(*ENB, 14.9.87*)

A. This question is more complicated than it looks and the answer needs care and attention. The student would benefit from formulating a plan of action before attempting an answer.

Client groups need to be identified first in order to be able to discuss the education given. Parentcraft should be geared to the needs of those in the class.

The student should note that she is asked to *discuss* the statement, therefore she needs to bring out problems both for and against providing a variety of classes, for example:

(i) grouping of different client groups;
(ii) when parentcraft education should begin
  school
  preconception
  antenatally
(iii) where classes should be carried out.

Q.9 (a) Describe the placenta and membranes at term. (20)
(b) Describe the functions of the mature placenta. (30)
(c) How may placental function be assessed during pregnancy? (50)

(*ENB, 7.7.86*) 100

A. Part (a) accounts for 20 per cent of the marks and allows the student to spend approximately nine minutes on her answer, which needs to be fairly brief but accurate. As the second part of the question asks for functions, a description of appearance, shape, size, weight, cord insertion and differentiation of maternal and fetal surfaces is required here.

Part (b) also needs to be fairly brief and could make use of headed paragraphs outlining the functions and how they fulfil all fetal requirements. The following headings could be used as a guide:

(i) respiratory function;
(ii) endocrine/hormonal function;
(iii) excretory function;
(iv) nutritive and glycogenic function;
(v) barrier/protection.

Part (c) accounts for the majority of the available marks so half the allotted time should be utilized here. The student would be expected to discuss the clinical skills of the midwife in assessing fetal growth and wellbeing, therefore indirectly assessing placental function. She should also recognize abnormalities in fetal growth and the need for referral for more intensive investigations. These could be discussed under the following headings:

(i) fetal heart recording;
(ii) ultrasound;
(iii) biochemical factors.

Sample questions and answers

Q.10 (a) **Define grande multiparity.** (10)
(b) **What potential problems place these women at risk?** (30)
(c) **Describe the management of these problems during pregnancy.** (60)

(ENB, 13.7.87) 100

A. This question is in three definte parts: part (a) carries a small proportion of the marks; part (b) a larger proportion, but the emphasis is on part (c).

Part (a): *definition* – this can only be loose as it tends to vary slightly but is a term generally applied to the woman who has given birth to four or more children.

Part (b): *potential problems* – these are probably best described under headings of

(i) antenatal
   anaemia,
   urinary tract infection,
   poor clinic attendance,
   intrauterine growth retardation,
   antepartum haemorrhage (both varieties),
   unstable lie,
   cord prolapse;
(ii) labour
   malpresentations and malpositions,
   hypotonic uterine contractions or precipitate labour,
   preterm labour,
   cephalopelvic disproportion,
   higher incidence of stillborn babies, congenital abnormality,
   postpartum haemorrhage;
(iii) postnatal
   lax pelvic floor muscles,
   tiredness and anaemia,
   varicose veins,
   thromboembolism,

infection;
(iv) other
older woman – hypertension,
obesity.

Part (c): *management:* – This should be related to the problems outlined in the previous section. As there is a lot of information to include it may be better to relate management to main reasons for complications occurring, in other words, relate unstable lie in pregnancy to management of this to minimize the risk of malpresentations and malpositions in labour, greater likelihood of cord prolapse, preterm labour, abnormal uterine action in labour and postpartum haemorrhage as they are all associated with lax abdominal and uterine muscles due to grande multiparity.

Work through other complications, grouping together where possible to save time and repetition.

Q.11 (a) **How could polyhydramnios be diagnosed?** (30)
(b) **What complications are associated with polyhydramnios?** (20)
(c) **Describe the immediate treatment of one of these conditions.** (50)

(*Queen Charlotte's Test Paper*) 100

A. As part (a) does not indicate whether it is acute or chronic polyhydramnios both varieties need to be included. The diagnosis can sometimes be confused with other conditions, such as multiple pregnancy and tumours, which can cause the uterus to appear larger than the expected size. Only specific signs that are found in polyhydramnios need to be emphasized.

For part (b) complications should be divided into:

(i) those conditions that cause polyhydramnios, such as:
congenital abnormality,
diabetes;

Sample questions and answers

(ii) those conditions that arise as a result of polyhydraminios, such as:
> excessive pressure symptoms,
> abnormal lie, presentation, position,
> ruptured membranes,
> cord prolapse,
> abruptio placentae,
> postpartum haemorrhage,
> amniotic fluid embolism.

For part (c) on treatment, the student should notice that there are two key words:

(i) *one* condition only to be described;
(ii) *your immediate* treatment indicates that the examiner is looking for the action of the midwife at a particular time, normally in an emergency situation.

Conditions that could be chosen are:

(i) prolapsed cord;
(ii) shoulder presentation;
(iii) abruptio placentae;
(iv) postpartum haemorrhage.

The action of the midwife is critical to the baby's survival in cord prolapse, if it is she who diagnoses it, whereas in the other conditions there is little she can do until medical aid arrives. This is a relevant point as this section accounts for half the available marks.

Q.12 (a) **Describe the changes that occur in the uterus during the first stage of labour.** (40)
(b) **How can the midwife assess that progress in normal in the first stage of labour?** (60)

(Adapted from ENB paper) 100

A. Part (a) should demonstrate the student's knowledge and understanding of the physiological changes that bring about effacement and dilatation of the cervix and lead to rupture of membranes and descent of the fetus. Included in the answer should be:

(i) effacement of the cervix;
(ii) dilatation of the cervix;
(iii) formation of retraction ring;
(iv) formation of bag of forewaters;
(v) rupture of membranes.

related to: fundal dominance, polarity, contraction and retraction of the myometrium in the upper uterine segment.

The assessment of progress in part (b) is the aspect the student would spend most time on (approximately twenty-five minutes). The answer should be in a logical sequence, and formulating a plan prior to answering the question is useful here. Stress that progress in the first stage of labour is assessed by the following:

(i) abdominal examination
   length, strength and frequency of contractions, lie and presentation, relating these to descent of the presenting part and what it would indicate;
(ii) vaginal examination
   degree of effacement, progressive dilatation of the cervix,
   application of the cervix to the presenting part,
   position of presenting part in relation to the ischial spines,
   attitude and flexion of fetal head,
   state of membranes.

The student should state how she would use the information to indicate normal progress and how both mother and fetus are coping with labour.

In this answer the student should indicate how frequently the above assessments are made and how she would relate the findings to the assessment of progress in *normal* labour. An explanation of the use of a partogram and cervicograph (with a diagram for preference) to give an overall impression of progress would be relevant here (Fig. 3).

Sample questions and answers

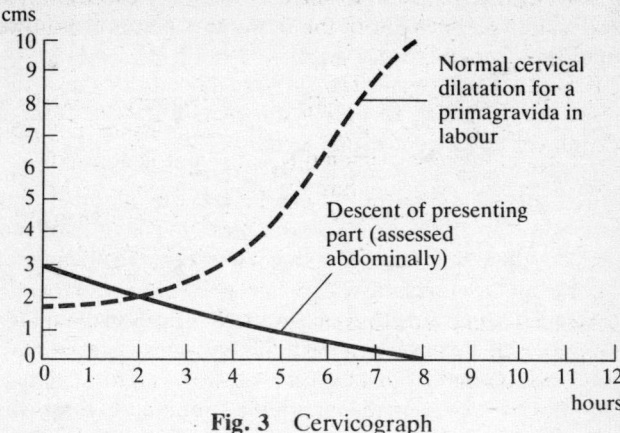

Fig. 3 Cervicograph

As the question states *normal* labour, it would be appropriate to mention the other recordings carried out on the mother and fetus (such as vital signs) and what the findings should be when labour is normal. This last part is not as important as the assessment of progress in this question and should not contain much elaboration.

Q.13 (a) **Outline the records that a midwife will make during the first stage of labour.** (20)
(b) **Describe how a midwife should recognize that the first stage of labour is progressing normallly.**

(80)

(*ENB, 8.9.86*)

100

A. Approximately nine minutes should be spent on the part (a) as it accounts for only 20 per cent of the marks. The student is asked for an *outline* of the records the midwife will make in the first stage of labour, so she does not need to go into great detail. It is important to outline baseline observations of vital signs, urinalysis, abdominal examination, vaginal examination and fetal heart rate. An indication of how often these are performed should be given and records kept.

If part (b) is read again it will be seen that most of the detailed information relating to normal progress in labour from the records will be included in that section.

The information required in part (b) is similar to that outlined in part (b) of question 12. As more marks are allocated to this part, however, the student's answer needs to contain a bit more detail. A definition of the first stage of labour and an outline of how the mother is coping with pain may be given, but this must be related to recognition of progress. Any deviation from normal in the aspects covered in this answer may indicate that progress is becoming *abnormal*.

Q.14 (a) Describe the anatomy of the pelvic floor. (30)
(b) List the causes of a third-degree tear. (20)
(c) How may the midwife reduce the risk of a third-degree tear in labour? (50)

(*Adapted from ENB paper*) 100

A. Part (a) deals with the anatomy of the pelvic floor, and the student would be unwise to attempt this question if she is not fully conversant with the pelvic floor musculature, as it accounts for almost a third of the marks.

Deep and superficial muscles should be named, and the different layers and the landmarks of their attachment described. The perineal body should also be described, together with function, blood, lymph and nerve supply. A clearly labelled diagram would be very helpful and may save a considerable amount of writing.

For part (b) define a third-degree tear before listing causes. Include in the answer:

(i) large baby;
(ii) large presenting part (for example persistent occipitoposterior position);

Sample questions and answers 55

(iii) extended, or poorly performed episiotomy;
(iv) poorly controlled delivery head/shoulders;
(v) narrow subpubic arch (especially if associated with a persistent occipitoposterior position)
(vi) previous third-degree tear;
(vii) impacted shoulders.

For part (c) the student should relate the midwife's ability to recognizing risk factors that predispose to a third-degree tear and how to minimize them. The examiner is also looking at the student's ability to further demonstrate her understanding of the pelvic floor, that is applying theoretical knowledge to the practical situation. The answer should bring out the following aspects:

(i) how knowledge of the anatomy and function of the pelvic floor may modify the midwife's management of the second stage of labour;
(ii) the benefits of one midwife only to give instructions in the second stage of labour;
(iii) building up the woman's confidence to obtain her cooperation (that is, education);
(iv) adequate pain relief in the period leading up to the second stage of labour will also enhance cooperation;
(v) appreciation of the presenting diameters, trying for example, to keep flexed if an occipitoanterior position;
(vi) constant assessment of the presenting part to identify abnormalities;
(vii) assessment of elasticity of the perineum – for example, 'buttonholing', slight bleeding, rigidity – may indicate the need for episiotomy;
(viii) adequate mediolateral episiotomy when indicated, for example, elective episotomy if there is a history of previous third-degree tear;
(ix) careful control of the presenting part before and after episiotomy;
(x) controlled delivery of shoulders.

All aspects highlighted should demonstrate the midwife's ability to take the appropriate action to minimize the risk of a third-degree tear; having identified the appropriate potential problem, what action should the student take to lessen the possibility of damage being sustained?

Q.15 (a) **Describe the anatomy of the perineal body.** (25)
(b) **Outline how the midwife may prevent or minimize:** (35)
  (i) **damage to the pelvic floor muscles in labour**
  (ii) **perineal pain during the early postnatal period.** (40)

(*ENB, 16.3.87*)   100

A. Part (a) requires a straightforward description of the anatomy of the perineal body and should include a diagram. This is difficult to do if the student has no specific knowledge. Do not make the mistake of describing the anatomy of the *whole* pelvic floor rather than the *perineal body* as requested.

Part (b) is divided into parts (i) and (ii) which are specifically directed to the *midwife's role* in preventing damage to the whole of the pelvic floor muscles in labour and management of perineal pain in the early postnatal period.

(i) Damage to the pelvic floor muscles in labour – this could be caused by:
    stretching of the deep muscles;
    laceration of the superficial, and sometimes deep, muscles.

The remainder of this part of the answer can then be devoted to prevention of this kind of damage occuring;

(1)   prevention of stretching of the deep muscles – particular attention should be paid to the following:
    assessment of onset of second stage of labour;
    avoiding 'pushing' for excessively long periods of time, especially likely with an occipitoposterior position;

assessment of progress in the second stage of labour; recognition that the second stage is becoming unduly prolonged, being aware that medical assistance may be required.

(2) prevention of lacerations – as well as those observations included above particular attention should be paid to:
> identification of the position of the presenting part;
> observing the perineum during descent of presenting part; is it stretching adequately, is episiotomy required?
> controlled delivery of presenting part and shoulders;
> any benefits to the use of perineal massage.

(ii) Perineal pain during the early postnatal period – the student should define what she considers to be the early postnatal period and confine her answer to the definition she has given. This should cover at least the first three days following delivery, and include in the answer prompt perineal repair following delivery.

The mother should be given explanation of what has happened and the reason for her experiencing pain and discomfort (knowledge will reduce both anxiety and pain).

Inspection of the perineum in the immediate post-partum period to assess oedema, bruising and exclude haematoma formation should be covered. The remainder of the answer could be divided into:
> advice given, sitting comfortably, feeding baby, chairs etc.;
> analgesia and other methods of reducing pain;
> daily care of the perineal area;
> recognition of abnormalities;
> mobility and hygiene;
> care of haemorrhoids, voiding urine, etc.

The student should explain why she considers these methods beneficial in reducing pain, and include any recent research relating to perineal problems in her answer.

Q.16 **A twenty-two-year-old primigravida, thirty-nine weeks pregnant, is admitted to a consultant unit following spontaneous onset of labour. Describe the management of her labour in anticipation of a normal delivery.**

100

(ENB, 13.7.87)

A. As this question is not divided into parts it could be written either in essay form or under headings. A plan is essential and the information given in the answer should follow some sensible order. As the question asks for management of labour in anticipation of a normal delivery the emphasis should be on the management of the first stage of labour and should include:

(i) admission
   general assessment,
   assessment of labour,
   specific observations, both maternal and fetal,
   expectations of labour and discussion of birth plan;
(ii) management in labour
   nursing care,
   maternal observations: frequency of recording and why they are carried out,
   fetal observations,
   assessment of progress in labour including vaginal examination,
   emotional support, both woman and partner,
   pain relief, ambulation,
   education,
   records,
   preparation for delivery.

Emphasis should be on the midwife's management of labour as a normal delivery is anticipated. The greater part of the answer

Sample questions and answers

should relate to how the midwife is recognizing that normal progress is taking place while ensuring that this is a satisfying and rewarding time for the woman and her partner.

Q.17 **A young healthy primigravida is admitted at forty-two weeks gestation to a consultant unit for induction of labour by amniotomy and intravenous oxytocin.**

(a) How should the midwife prepare the parents for these procedures? (50)

(b) Describe the care which should be given until labour is established. (50)

(*ENB, 12.1.87*) 100

As this question is divided into two equal parts half the available time should be spent on each part of the answer. A plan is really essential to this answer.

In part (a) the student should note that she is dealing with a young healthy primigravida. This implies that no abnormalities are anticipated, and the answer should reflect this – to date no specific problems have been identified, and the induction is being performed only because the pregnancy is postmature and could be considered as a relatively straightforward procedure. The procedure is not completely risk-free, but this should come out in tackling part (b).

A primigravid woman will have no previous experience of induction of labour to draw on. Information-giving and support is very important to ensure that the woman understands fully why the procedure is to be performed, how it will be performed, and what the anticipated outcome will be.

Discussing preparing the *parents* for these procedures gives some idea that the role of the midwife as an educator as well as provider of emotional support for both partners is an important factor in this answer.

Specific information in this part should include:

(i) an explanation, to both partners, of what the procedures are and why they are being performed, with an outline of subsequent management and expected outcome.

(ii) an explanation of why it is important to prepare the couple fully:

what emotional support can be provided for them? What measures could be employed to allay their anxieties? How might their expectations of labour be altered?

(iii) the physical care likely to be performed prior to amniotomy and consideration of the administration of intravenous oxytocin.

Part (b) is much more factual although emotional support must not be ignored. It could be assumed that the care to be given is from the time that amniotomy is performed and intravenous oxytocin commenced. An explanation of what established labour is would be helpful.

Some overlap of information given will probably occur although this should be kept to a minimum. It is important to read the question carefully and detail care given until labour is established. This care should include:

(i) general physical care, routine observations and care of the bladder;
(ii) specific observations of maternal and fetal wellbeing, how often they will be carried out and why they are being performed:

observations following artificial rupture of membranes, care of an oxytocic infusion,
monitoring of maternal wellbeing,
monitoring of fetal wellbeing.

The student should bring out possible dangers to the mother and fetus associated with these two procedures, stressing emotional support for both partners. How would she ensure general comfort and hygiene? Recording of information gained should be included.

In this question an assessment is being made by the examiners

Sample questions and answers

of: (1) the student's knowledge of the role of the midwife and her ability to provide safe, effective care while ensuring that emotional support is given to both partners throughout; and (2) the limitations of practice (when to refer for consultation).

Q.18 (a) Describe how a midwife would perform an emergency breech delivery in the absence of medical help, giving reasons for her actions. (70)
(b) Outline the complications of vaginal breech delivery which might affect the newborn baby. (30)

(ENB, 4.11.86)   100

A. This question is designed to assess the student's ability to cope with what is luckily becoming an increasingly rare situation – vaginal breech delivery. It is also designed to test the student's knowledge of the mechanism through which the baby presenting by the breech must traverse, and the implications for the fetus in part (b).

In part (a) it is important to specify that the aim is to prevent physical trauma to mother and baby and this should be considered during the mechanism described. Points to be considered include:

(i) *Preparation for the delivery:*
equipment for resuscitation,
delivery pack,
lithotomy position if possible,
confirmation of onset of the second stage of labour, by vaginal examination, to ensure that the fetal body is not pushed through a partially dilated cervical os.

(ii) *Actual delivery:*
bladder empty
reduce trauma to bladder,
aid descent of fetus by improving contractions;
episiotomy when perineum is distended to enable manoeuvres as appropriate for delivering the limbs and head;

describe delivery of lower limbs, umbilical cord, body, arms, neck and head, bringing out the importance of why you are undertaking various procedures and how this prevents undue trauma to mother and baby;

oxytocic drugs: when are they likely to be administered with a breech delivery, and how it differs from normal;

briefly state how to conduct the third stage (completion of delivery) as for any other labour.

In part (b) a logical sequence would be to work through labour as complications are then less likely to be forgotten. Note that the question specifies *vaginal* breech delivery. Complications included should cover:

(i) the greater likelihood of cord prolapse due to poorly fitting presenting part;
(ii) pushing before the cervix is fully dilated with implications for the baby;
(iii) physical trauma to the baby occuring during delivery:
    fractured femur,
    abdominal organ damage (adrenals, liver, spleen),
    fractured clavical, humerus,
    fractured neck,
    cerebral damage,
    facial palsies,
    generalized oedema and bruising;
(iv) hypoxia
    as secondary to cord compression,
    in a prolonged second stage;
(v) hypothermia;
(vi) increased perinatal mortality and morbidity as a result of above factors.

Sample questions and answers

Q.19 (a) List the factors predisposing to primary postpartum haemorrhage. (20)
(b) Outline the measures that should be taken by a midwife to reduce the risk of this occurring. (30)
(c) In the event of such a haemorrhage occurring at home, what action should be taken by the midwife?
(50)
———
(*Adapted from ENB paper*) 100
———

A. A brief introduction should be given to include a definition of primary postpartum haemorrhage, the incidence of its occurrence and the effect it could have on the mother (refer to avoidable maternal mortality).

Part (a) asks for a *list* only and could be divided into:

(i) failure of the uterus to contract – enlarge on predisposing factors;
(ii) trauma – again enlarge;
(iii) incidental factors – give examples.

Part (b) asks for an *outline* only of the measures that could be taken by a midwife to reduce such a risk and should include:

(i) the importance of antenatal care with particular reference to haemoglobin estimations and diet;
(ii) the importance of correct place of confinement for those women most at risk;
(iii) the skilled management of all stages of labour;
(iv) care of the bladder in labour and during delivery;
(v) the request for the presence of an obstetrician for the delivery for those women most at risk (for example, previous postpartum haemorrhage);
(vi) the use of oxytocic drugs.

Part (c) carries 50 per cent of the marks and should therefore carry a full account of the action a midwife would take if confronted with this emergency in the home. The examiner is looking at the student's ability to deal with an emergency situation while maintaining safety. Events must be given in a logical sequence to demonstrate her ability to cope in such a situation.

Information in the answer should cover:

(i) immediate emergency measures to control haemorrhage while sending for urgent medical aid (in other words, emergency obstetric flying squad);
(ii) the use of an oxytocic drug to control haemorrhage;
(iii) the delivery of the placenta and membranes if still *in situ* – examine placenta and membranes for completeness if already delivered;
(iv) estimating and saving of blood loss; treating for shock;
(v) the taking and recording of appropriate observations as guide to maternal wellbeing;
(vi) care of the bladder;
(vii) the reassurance of the mother and her family;
(viii) the early acquisition of the appropriate blood samples of crossmatching and haemoglobin levels;
(ix) possible completion of consent to anaesthetic form;
(x) the technique of bimanual compression should other methods to control haemorrhage fail.

The short conclusion could include a reiteration of the midwife's prompt action while waiting for medical assistance and the value of efficient teamwork in such an emergency when assistance arrives.

Q.20 Describe the care a midwife will give to mother and her baby during the twenty-eight days following delivery. 100

(ENB, 8.9.86)

A. This is a fairly straightforward 100 per cent question where the examiner will be expecting a description of the midwife's role in the postnatal period. This role would be the same whether the mother and baby were in hospital or at home.

As the question specifies both mother and baby, the student should include the midwife's responsibility to both to an equal

Sample questions and answers

degree. This type of question requires a definite answer plan as time is limited and there is much essential information to include. Do not stray from the point or 'waffle'.

The answer should start with a *brief* outline of care following delivery and prior to transfer to the postnatal area. Specific information should be given on:

(i) statutory duties of the midwife in providing postnatal care (in other words, care must be provided up to ten days and may extend to twenty-eight days if necessary);
(ii) general physical care of mother including daily observations and examination with an explanation of why they are performed;
(iii) general physical care of the baby including daily observations and examination with an explanation of why they are performed;
(iv) establishment of feeding;
(v) education of mother and family;
(vi) assessment of maternal care of baby (both physical and emotional);
(vii) provision of emotional support;
(viii) individualization of care;
(ix) record-keeping and documentation;
(x) advice given to mother/family at the time of discharge from the midwife's care (including family planning);
(xi) liaison with other primary health care personnel responsible for carrying out follow-up care;
(xii) an example of instances in which the midwife may wish to extend her visits beyond ten days.

Bring out the unique role of the midwife in providing the care described.

Q.21 Describe the care a midwife should provide for a mother and her baby during the first twenty-eight days following delivery. 100

(*ENB, 12.1.87*)

A. This question is almost identical to question **20** and could be tackled in exactly the same way or, if a different approach is required headings could be used.

Again, the student needs to decide where to begin the care. It would seem reasonable to begin with care immediately the baby is born, but because the question asks for the first twenty-eight days, there is no time to discuss in detail resuscitation and the first examination of the newborn. Care of the *mother* should begin with completion of the third stage and repair of the perineum.

Headings could encompass the following:

Mother	*Baby*
physical care	routine care
emotional care	screening tests
statutory records	follow-up
education	
communication	

Q.22 Describe in detail the observations the midwife will make on the mother in the first week following delivery and why these observations are made.

100

A. This, again, is very similar to questions **20** and **21** but it should be noted that the question asks specifically for observations the midwife will make on the *mother* and only during the first seven days following delivery.

This question is asking the student to consider what, for her, is a very common procedure, and to look at the reasoning behind observations made in the first week postnatally.

The observations should start immediately following the third stage of labour and could conveniently be divided into two parts:

(i) first twenty-four hours;
(ii) twenty-four hours to the end of the first week.
(i) *First twenty-four hours*
   The emphasis would be on assessing how the woman has

coped with the physical act of childbearing, for example
   detection of haemorrhage,
   pre-eclampsia,
   haematoma formation, etc.,
in relation to information in the labour ward notes.
Psychological adaptation to motherhood should also be considered.

(ii) *Twenty-four hours to the end of the first week*
The emphasis would be less on the physical act of childbearing and more on the return of the body to the non-pregnant state and the physical and emotional adjustment of parenting, for example:
   general wellbeing,
   breasts, feeding regime,
   involution of the uterus, lochia,
   thromboembolic problems,
   bladder/bowels,
   perineum,
   sleep pattern, early detection of postnatal depression,
   attitude and confidence with baby,
   emotional state,
   postnatal exercises.

To provide a well-balanced answer to this question, a full explanation should be given as to why all the above are being considered.

Q.23 (a) **Outline the physical and emotional preparation for a mother for Caesarean section.** (30)
(b) **List the emotional problems that may arise following any Caesarean section.** (20)
(c) **Describe briefly the midwife's role in caring for a mother in the first week following Caesarean section.** (50)

(*ENB, 14.9.87*)   100

A. Part (a) is quite straightforward and should be divided into:

(i) physical preparation, including skin preparation, bladder care, consent for operation and prevention of Mendelson's syndrome;
(ii) emotional preparation, including reassurance and a visit to the special care baby unit if possible.

Part (b) accounts for 20 per cent of the marks, and the student should note that she is only required to list *emotional* problems. These might include:

(i) feeling of failure as labour has not been experienced;
(ii) fear of outcome;
(iii) lose of body image;
(iv) separation from baby, etc.

A qualifying sentence for each item listed would enhance the answer.

Part (c) should take half the available time as it accounts for 50 per cent of the marks. The answer should include:

(i) communication and education;
(ii) physical care – include *all* normal postnatal care but be brief;
    care of wound and abdomen generally, for example, bowel sounds,
    care of intravenous infusion,
    care of bladder,
    ambulation,
    help with feeding,
    analgesia,
    prevention of deep vein thrombosis and other complications;
emotional support.

Sample questions and answers

Q.24 What care and advice may be given to a (40)
primigravida by the midwife in order to promote
and support successful breast-feeding:

    (a) during pregnancy
    (b) during the first ten days after birth? (50)
    (c) What help is available to a mother who is
breast-feeding once she has been discharged from
the midwife's care? (10)

(ENB, 4.11.86)   100

A. Questions related to feeding, both breast and artificial, are common in examination papers. It is really asking the student to examine her practice and the practice of midwives with whom she has worked in relation to promoting breast-feeding.

Part (a), because of the weighting, warrants almost half the time to be spent on it (approximately twenty minutes). It should include such aspects as:

(i) accurate information for the couple pertaining to the breast changes in pregnancy and an outline of the physiology of lactation and correct 'fixing' of the baby.
(ii) discussing honestly any fears/hesitations the woman has;
(iii) rectifying 'old wives' tales';
(iv) physical preparation of the breasts to prepare for breast-feeding;
(v) dietary advice;
(vi) discussion of the women's postnatal 'routine', demand feeding and the practicality of breast-feeding.

Part (b) must be a continuation of part (a) together with addressing the practical issues directly involved in breast-feeding such as:

(i)   fixing the baby;
(ii)   demand feeding;
(iii)   prevention of engorgement, sore nipples;
(iv)   removing the baby with little trauma;
(v)   positions for feeding;

(vi) care of breasts;
(vii) information pertaining to 'crying baby'
(viii) going out, expression of breast milk;
(ix) communication with the community midwife when discharged home;
(x) consistent advice, therefore contact with as few midwives as possible;
(xi) importance of care plan.

Aim to build up the woman's confidence in caring for her own baby.

Part (c) requires the student to be aware of other personnel, both medical and non-medical, who may be of help to the mother, for example:

National Childbirth Trust;
La Lèche League;
health visitors.

Q.25 (a) **How may a midwife recognize postnatal depression?** (30)
(b) **List the factors predisposing to depression during the postnatal period.** (20)
(c) **What help and support may the midwife give to a depressed mother and her family in the twenty-eight days following delivery?** (50)

(ENB, 14.9.87) 100

A. This is a straightforward question that should present no problems. When answering part (a) it would be helpful to differentiate between postnatal depression and postnatal 'blues'. It may be easier to tackle this part of the question by considering:

(i) what the mother herself may complain of, such as insomnia, persistent anxiety over baby, weepiness, etc.;
(ii) what the family may notice, such as acting out of

character, excessive mood swings, apathy, obsessional behaviour with baby, etc.;
(iii) what the midwife may notice in addition to all the above, such as excessive number of questions from mother, general inability to cope, failure of baby to thrive, mother unkempt, house excessively untidy, etc.

Part (b) asks for a list of predisposing factors. Consideration should be given to:

(i) previous history;
(ii) physical factors likely to affect mental state;
(iii) psychological factors;
(iv) factors relating to baby, for example, handicap, stillbirth, etc.

Part (c) looks at the midwife's ability to give positive, practical help to a depressed mother in the first twenty-eight days postnatally. Reference should be made to what the student has written in parts (a) and (b) to identify some of the areas where help with practical aspects and additional support can be given. The mother's emotional, physical and mental state should be assessed regularly, plus her ability to care for the baby. Highlight the benefits of continuity of care with one midwife in recognizing changes early and taking appropriate action to relieve these, building up a rapport with the mother and her family. Allow the mother time to talk about her problems and anxieties and express her fears – in other words, be sensitive to the mother's needs, giving additional emotional support and help.

Educate the family to be of assistance in providing positive support.

Call in other agencies, such as general practitioner, health visitor, social workers, psychiatrist for additional assistance.

Bring out the role of the midwife in providing holistic care for both mother and family to try and prevent depression becoming more severe.

Q.26 (a) Describe a healthy full-term baby on the day
following delivery. (40)
(b) How would you teach a mother to recognize
that her baby is making satisfactory progress in
the first week of life? (60)

(ENB, 7.7.86) 100

A. Although this appears to be a straightforward question students frequently fail to read the question properly and describe the *examination* of the baby following delivery. It is important to note in part (a) that the question is asking for a description of the healthy full-term baby on the *day following* delivery, not *at* delivery.

Included in the answer of part (a) a description of the following would be expected:

(i) normal weight and measurements range;
(ii) appearance – colour, muscle tone, condition of skin, etc.;
(iii) behaviour – ability to maintain temperature, sleeping, reflexes, feeding, cry, activity, etc.;
(iv) elimination of waste products;
(v) condition of umbilical cord.

In part (b) the key aspects to note are:

(i) *teach* the mother;
(ii) satisfactory *progress*;
(iii) *first week* of life (the first seven days)

In this answer it is important for the student to indicate not only *what* she would teach the mother but *how* she would teach it. As with any teaching it is necessary to assess the level of existing knowledge and work from that point. Bring out in the answer that it is important to pitch teaching at the correct level for the particular mother being taught. Consider different methods of teaching – for instance, on a one-to-one basis, or group teaching.

The environment in which teaching is to take place also needs

Sample questions and answers

to be briefly considered as well as making the mother feel comfortable and unhurried and able to ask questions. This information could take approximately a third of the time allocated to this part. The subsequent two-thirds should include the content of what the mother is taught, for example:

(i) normal behaviour – response to stimuli (noise, touch, cry);
(ii) normal behaviour – feeding, sleeping patterns, etc.;
(iii) weight variations, normal weight gain;
(iv) explanation of normal elimination patterns;
(v) information gained from observation – skin, mouth, stools etc.

The student will realize that she is again concentrating on the role of the midwife. The question is less worrying if the normal, everyday teaching role in the postnatal area, and aspects felt to be important for physical and emotional development, are considered.

Q.27 A full-term breast-fed baby has a small weight loss on the fourth day and a further weight loss on the sixth day of life.
(a) What information should the midwife obtain to determine possible causes for this weight loss? (50)
(b) What action should the midwife take? (50)

(*ENB, 14.9.87*) 100

A. The statement at the beginning of this question spells out that a *full-term*, *breast-fed* baby is being considered, therefore care must be taken not to include irrelevant information.

The amount of weight loss is not defined; however, from the information required by the examiners in part (a) the student must state what she would consider to be an abnormal weight loss and confine her answer mainly to this aspect.

(a) *Information obtained by the midwife* should cover the following:

(i) Feeding
   reduction in demand,
   reduction in supply,
   reduction through mechanical difficulty;
(ii) Presence of infection;
(iii) general health of baby;
(iv) undetected congenital abnormality (for example, cardiac disease);
(v) information related to mother's general health;
(vi) information related to mother's emotional health;
(vii) related social factors;
(viii) elimination of human error with weight recording.

When considering any of these factors it is important to highlight the significance of the information obtained to give a balanced answer.

(b) Part (b) is concerned with the midwife's *subsequent actions* to combat or overcome the problems encountered. These could be discussed under the same heading identified in part (a), special consideration being given to the need for referral for medical advice and subsequent care.

Further discussion could take place on the midwife's role in respect of:

(i) supervision of feeding;
(ii) education;
(iii) counselling;
(iv) support and reassurance;
(v) documentation of observations and findings;
(vi) communication with other health professionals.

Care should be taken not to overlap too much on part (a) as this makes the answer repetitious.

Q.28 Describe the care of a preterm baby born at thirty-four weeks gestation.

(*ENB, 13.7.87*)

Sample questions and answers

A. This question is not divided into parts and therefore could be answered either in essay form or under headings.

A baby born at thirty-four weeks gestation may encounter none of the problems associated with a preterm baby, or may suffer from one or all of the complications of prematurity. In view of this optimum place for providing nursing care should be considered.

It would be reasonable to first describe principles of care for any preterm baby with an explanation of each principle. Then, consider briefly care required for any individual complications of prematurity likely to develop.

The introduction could include:

(i) implications of a preterm birth both in the short-term and long-term, regarding mortality and morbidity;
(ii) the effects that such a birth may have on maternal/infant attachment;
(iii) the possible problems involved with family integration, a general statement on the problems involved in the care of such an infant.

The body of the answer should include:

(i) *general care of a preterm infant*
place of nursing and general nursery environment, such as temperature;
daily care;
nutrition – calorific requirements, method of feeding with reasons for choice;
maintenance of temperature;
prevention of infection;
observations and use of any appropriate specialized equipment;
recording of all relevant information on care plan or in another appropriate place.
(ii) *Specific complications*
jaundice – briefly describe nursing care, including observations;

respiratory distress – importance of achieving correct oxygenation of infant, methods of administering oxygen. Reiterate importance of general nursing care;

hypothermia – methods of achieving normal temperature;

hypoglycaemia – methods for returning the glycogenic state to normal;

infection – prevention of cross-infection.

A paragraph can be included stating that there are many more problems the preterm baby may encounter, but the above are the most common.

For a conclusion:

(i) reiterate the importance of skilled care and the need to care for the parents as well as the baby;
(ii) stress communication with other professionals and follow-up care.

Q.29 Following a period of unsatisfactory intrauterine growth, a baby is born at thirty-eight weeks gestation with an Apgar score of eight. (40)
(a) Describe how fetal growth and wellbeing may have been assessed during pregnancy.
(b) Discuss the care that may be necessary for the baby during the first week of life. (60)

(ENB, 16.3.87) 100

A. This is a question that relates events in the antenatal period to care required in the postnatal period. The initial statement indicates that the baby is growth-retarded, born at term and in good condition.

Part (a) gives a straightforward description of fetal growth and wellbeing during preganancy. It is important to remember that intrauterine growth retardation is initially suspected on clinical examination, so commence with routine clinical observations and work up to the more specific investigations. An explanation of the significance of each investigation covered should be given. Specific investigations might include the following:

(i) ultrasound assessment of fetal growth;
(ii) placental hormone assays;
(iii) use of 'Cardiff' kick charts;
(iv) cardiotocography for assessing fetal wellbeing;
(v) other tests, for example, abdominal girth measurement, exclusion of other abnormalities, and other blood tests.

Part (b) asks for *discussion*. Care would commence from the moment of delivery which should be in a consultant unit. With the known antenatal history it would be appropriate for the paediatrician to be present at delivery. Although the question gives the Apgar score at delivery it does not give any indication of *size* of the baby. Discussion should centre on the most appropriate place to nurse the baby (such as transfer to special care baby unit, transitional care, or care on the postnatal ward).

Care discussed should include both routine care, as for any baby, plus specific care in relation to growth retardation, for example:

(i) initial care on the labour ward;
(ii) routine care of the newborn in the first week of life;
(iii) significance of type, method and time of feeding, calorific requirements;
(iv) significance of regular estimations of serum glucose levels;
(v) the importance of the thermoneutral environment;
(vi) the extra observations a growth-retarded baby may need in relation to condition of the baby;
(vii) the possible effect of a growth-retarded infant on maternal/infant attachment;
(viii) counselling for parents.

Q.30 (a) List the causes of jaundice in the newborn. (20)
(b) Describe the care of a baby with hyperbilirubinaemia occurring within twenty-four hours of birth. (80)

(*Adapted from ENB paper*)

100

A. In the part (a) it is insufficient to give a straightforward list of causes. An outline explanation of the pathology is also necessary, for example:

(i) physiological jaundice;
(ii) haemolytic jaundice
  rhesus incompatability,
  ABO incompatability,
  abnormal red blood cells,
  other antibodies;
(iii) infection;
(iv) galactosaemia;
(v) breast milk jaundice;
(vi) obstructive jaundice.

The commonest causes should always be listed first followed by less commonly seen conditions.

In part (b) it is important to stress that hyperbilirubinaemia occurring during the first twenty-four hours of life is pathological *not* physiological, the most likely cause being due to haemolytic disease. A definition of hyperbilirubinaemia should be given with a statement to the effect that the significance of an abnormally high serum bilirubin level is dependent upon the gestational age, weight, age in days and general wellbeing of the baby. An example would be appropriate, followed by a care plan for the baby with haemolytic disease.

The management for any baby with hyperbilirubinaemia is, in part, directed towards the prevention of encephalopathy (kernicterus). Included in the answer should be the complete care given to the baby; points discussed should include:

(i) optimum place of care;

(ii)   general care;
(iii) specific observations;
(iv)   investigations undertaken;
(v)   monitoring of serum bilirubin levels;
(vi)   use of phototherapy;
(vii) exchange transfusion – although not always required the procedure should be described with care during and after it;
(viii) use of albumin;
(ix)   feeding regime/calories;
(x)   record-keeping;
(xi)   explanation to and counselling of parents;
(xii) communication with relevant health professionals regarding consequences;
(xiii) follow-up.

Q.31 Prevention of infection is of prime importance in reducing neonatal mortality and morbidity.
   (a) Describe the defences against infection which the healthy, full-term baby has at birth. (25)
   (b) What may the midwife do to minimize the risks of infection and cross-infection during the first ten days of life? (25)

   (ENB, 9.9.86)   100

A. Part (a) of this question should occupy about ten minutes of time allotted as it accounts for a quarter of the marks. It is very important to bear in mind that this question refers to a *healthy, full-term* baby, not growth-retarded or preterm.

A straight description should be given of both specific and non-specific defences:

(i)   non-specific
      skin – barrier if unbroken,
      phagocytosis by macrophages,
      inflammatory response;

(ii) specific
> antibody response to specific antigenic stimuli,
> cellular immunity,
> humoral immunity and IgM.

Part (b) could be tackled as separate entities, (i) infection and (ii) cross-infection, or the two discussed together. It should be noted that the question specifies the first ten days of life and the role of the midwife in minimizing infection; this would also include her role as educator and role model.

Some consideration should be given to this answer from delivery through to the immediate postnatal period and then up to the tenth day. Points covered could include discussion on the midwife's role in providing:

(i)   clean environment;
(ii) importance of hygiene and handwashing;
(iii) use of separate equipment for each baby;
(iv) use of sterile equipment for some procedures;
(v)   adequate amount of clean linen, safe disposal and used linen;
(vi) sterilizing of feeding equipment, plus correct usage;
(vii) clean areas where baby is to be placed;
(viii) personal hygiene of staff, parents, visitors;
(ix) overcrowding, nursery space, 'rooming in';
(x)   benefits of breast-feeding in relation to antibodies;
(xi) education of parents on care of baby, hygiene, etc.;
(xii) early discharge home to minimize cross-infection;
(xiii) prompt detection of infection (daily examination of baby) and early treatment;
(xiv) protection of baby from those with colds, infections etc.;
(xv) isolation of baby if necessary.

Sample questions and answers 81

Q.32 Severe fetal abnormality has been diagnosed during the antenatal period.
(a) How may fetal abnormality be diagnosed antenatally? (40)
(b) What care and support can the midwife give to assist parents whose severely abnormal baby is not expected to live more than a few days?

(60)

(*ENB, 12.1.87*) 100

A. In part (a) a factual answer is required as the question asks *how* fetal abnormality may be diagnosed in the antenatal period. The examiner will be expecting details of the importance of:

(i) history given at initial booking and subsequently;
(ii) clinical examination;
(iii) diagnostic tests available.

When discussing diagnostic methods for identifying fetal abnormality the commonest methods should be dealt with first (such as detailed ultrasound scan, amniocentesis) then less common investigations (such as fetoscopy). Newer techniques (such as chorionic villus sampling, CVS) could be included, although it is important to stress that these tests may increase the risk of miscarriage with a potentially normal fetus.

Part (b) requires the student to bring out the full role of the midwife in providing all the support necessary over this difficult period. Care should be taken to to stress positive aspects of the midwife's role, for example:

(i) one midwife designated to care for the woman;
(ii) encouraging contact with/use of name/handling baby;
(iii) photographs of baby;
(iv) encouraging parents to express feelings;
(v) adequate, honest explanation of what is happening and what is being done and whom?
(vi) what other resources/support groups are available;

(vii) what normal care will be required (statutory duties of the midwife);
(viii) counselling available;
(ix) notifying general practitioner/health visitor;
(x) allowing unlimited access to baby/involve extended family if parents wish;
(xi) how much care the parents themselves can give;
(xii) support of other family members;
(xiii) emotional support;
(xiv) preparation for subsequent events.

Q.33 **(a) Define stillbirth.** (10)
(b) List the predisposing causes of stillbirth. (20)
(c) Outline the statutory duties of the midwife when a stillbirth occurs. (20)
(d) Describe how the midwife may contribute to the emotional support of the bereaved parents. (50)

(*ENB, 9.9.86*) 100

A. If parts (a), (b) and (c) are not adequately known (especially the definition and statutory duties of the midwife) it would be unwise to attempt this question.

The definition of a stillbirth should be accurate and complete as cited in the UKCC Midwife's Code of Practice (1986), p.11. Predisposing factors should be listed, perhaps with a few examples. It may assist the presentation if the list is divided into fetal, placental and maternal causes. Commonest causes should be highlighted, first, followed by less common causes being listed last.

An *outline* of statutory duties is asked for, so explanations should be kept to the point. Cover notification, registration, in what circumstances the midwife may need to issue a stillbirth certificate and involvement of the supervisor of midwives. Refer again, to the UKCC Midwife's Code of Practice (1986), p.9–11.

Part (d) asks specifically for emotional support and is confined to the bereaved parents. The majority of the answer should relate to post-delivery care, especially as the previous section states 'when a stillbirth occurs'. However, it is important not to ignore the role of the midwife in the preparation of the parents before birth as this may relate directly to the amount of emotional support required after the stillbirth. If the parents know what to expect this may go a long way to alleviate some of the emotional trauma.

Part of the answer should indicate that the amount of support required may relate to when the stillbirth occurs, in other words has it been diagnosed, or is it unexpected? The answer could be broken down into emotional support required:

(i) before birth – includes communication, answering questions and preparation for labour (for example, how labour may be managed, holding baby);
(ii) during labour – communication, explanation of situation, being aware and sensitive to the parents needs;
(iii) following delivery – seeing and holding baby and what this achieves, naming baby, benefits of a photograph, allowing parents time together with their baby, a clear explanation of the legal formalities that follow a stillbirth needs to be given a part of emotional care, where to nurse the mother post-delivery, flexibility with visiting, checking on family support available, continuity of care to avoid conflicting information, advice, etc., allowing access to baby as necessary, providing information on support organizations, communication with other professionals like to come into contact with the family, sensitivity with regard to funeral arrangements, explanation of follow-up care for this couple.

These are all some of the points the student may wish to consider for her answer on providing emotional support. She may like to bring out the value of some of the work done by others (such as Esther Rantzen) highlighting how we can further improve our support.

Q.34 (a) Describe the factors that may lead to child abuse. (50)
 (b) List the signs of child abuse. (20)
 (c) What action should the midwife take if she suspects a child is being illtreated or neglected? (30)

(*ENB, 16.3.87*) 100

A. Although it is not specifically asked for in this question, a definition of what child abuse is would be useful to set the parameters of the answer. When answering this question it is important to look at wider issues as it is often other family members that are abusing or involved; in other words, the question does not specify a particular mother or baby but obviously relates to a family to which the midwife is giving professional care.

Part (a) asks for a description of the factors that lead to child abuse and accounts for 50 per cent of the available marks. The factors could be divided into sections in several different ways, therefore it would be a good idea to make a plan first to gather the information and decide how it is going to be presented.

The student may like to consider factors leading to child abuse under social circumstances, or those related to the effects of pregnancy and childbearing on existing circumstances, for example:

(i) *Social circumstances*
marital problems,
financial problems,
unemployment,
single parent,
large family,
drug/alcohol abuse,
poor home conditions,
multitudinous factors.

(ii) *Effect of pregnancy*
antenatal: pregnancy unplanned, unwanted, not partner's baby,

labour: unrealistic expectations, difficult labour, baby wrong sex,

postnatal: failure of mother/baby interaction, baby ill/separation, crying baby, inadequate mother, etc.

In part (b) a list is asked for with perhaps an initial clarifying sentence. Very often the injuries related do not tie up with events explained.

Similarly, in part (c) it is important to recognize that the newborn baby is not necessarily the subject of abuse, it could be other siblings. The question also implies that while ill treatment and neglect may not be life-threatening, at this point in time some immediate action needs to be taken by the midwife.

Each health authority will have its own guidelines for dealing with suspected cases of child abuse and these should be followed. It is important to bring out some of the following issues in the answer:

(i) involvement of the supervisor of midwives;
(ii) involvement of other health professionals, especially general practitioner, health visitor and social worker;
(iii) documentation of why the midwife suspects illtreatment or neglect;
(iv) how the midwife could provide positive help to this particular family;
(v) in the rare event of no other professional person being available involvement of other bodies (for example, police).

Q.35 What factors should be taken into consideration by the midwife when discussing the choice of contraceptive methods with a recently delivered mother?
(ENB, 13.7.87) 100

A. This is a 100 per cent question and it is therefore important that the student plans her answer to include all aspects to the question, and that she also considers carefully how she will present her material. In this instance it could be in essay form without headings, in which case the paragraphs will divide the work, or under headings for each area introduced.

The key words in this question are:

factors, consideration, midwife, discussing, choice, contraceptive method and **recently delivered mother.**

The introduction should include:
(i) significance of the words 'recently delivered mother';
(ii) what the student sees as the role of the midwife in this case;
(iii) why family planning is important;
(iv) the rights of women regarding family planning.

The body of the work should include:
(i) *physiological and pathological changes in the postnatal period:*
    reasons for possible change of contraceptive,
    changes in the uterus, cervix and vagina,
    changes in levels of oestrogen and progesterone and their signficance in relation to contraception and the newly delivered mother,
    psychological reaction to pregnancy,
    significance of any perineal injury,
    significance of a raised blood pressure, diabetes, varicose veins etc.

(ii) *lactation*
    The possibility or otherwise of using breast-feeding as a means of contraception,
    research on the action of breast-feeding on ovarian function, significance of weaning on contraception.

(iii) *sociological factors*
    the mother's views on contraception,
    her religious persuasions and any restrictions this may impose on her choice,
    her partner's feelings about contraception and any problems these may create,
    Her age and marital status and any problems this may present.

Sample questions and answers

(iii) *advantages and disadvantages of each suitable method* – these should be discussed in relation to the physiological changes taking place and already outlined. Methods covered should include:
  barrier methods,
  combined oral contraception, progesterone pill,
  intrauterine contraceptive devices (IUCDs),
  postpartum sterilization, vasectomy.
  natural and Billing's method should be discussed to highlight the difficulty of using these two methods in the immediate postpatum period.

The conclusion should briefly recap the student's answer stressing the salient points discussed in each paragraph.

Q.36 (a) **List the types of drugs which may be carried by midwives working in the community.** (15)
(b) **Describe how community midwives may:**
  obtain and store controlled drugs (20)
  administer and record the giving of controlled drugs (15)
  arrange for the destruction of controlled drugs. (10)
(c) **Discuss the value of pethidine as a suitable analgesic drug for mother during labour.** (40)

(*ENB, 8.9.86*)   100

A. This question is basically broken down into three parts and is designed to test the student's knowledge relating to the administration of mainly controlled drugs in her sphere of practice.

The important words to note in part (a) are: *list*, *types of drugs* and *midwives/community*. A simple list of the recommended different *categories* of drugs specific to community midwives is required (refer to UKCC Midwives Code of Practice, 1986, p.5). There is probably sufficient time to give an example for each category, for example analgesic: paracetamol, pethidine.

Part (b) relates to the obtaining, storage, administration,

recording and destruction of *controlled drugs* – again related to community practice. This requires a factual answer giving specific knowledge. As different community midwifery practices may vary slightly the student may be advised to consider what is common practice in the community to which she is attached. Specific recommendations, however, are laid down in both the UKCC Midwives Code of Practice, 1986, (p.5) and the UKCC Midwives Rules, 1986 (p.15) and the student should be completely conversant with these. Parts (a) and (b) combined account for 60 per cent of the available marks.

In part (c) the student should particularly note the words *discuss* and *value*. The examiners have stated very clearly that it is the use of pethidine as an analgesic drug in labour that should be discussed; students should be able to argue its benefits and contraindications. This should include beneficial and adverse factors to mother and fetus. The current view held by practitioners, in the unit where you have undertaken your midwifery training, on the use of pethidine in labour could be discussed here with any relevant personal comments that you may wish to include.

Current research findings could be of value in this answer.

Q.37 Explain the UKCC Midwives Rules in relation to: (25)
  (a) **notification of intention to practise**
  (b) **duty to record the administration of drugs** (25)
  (c) **duty to keep records** (25)
  (d) **calling medical assistance in an emergency** (25)

(*ENB, 12.1.87*) 100

A. Each section carries a quarter of the available marks allowing approximately 10 minutes for each component.

The examiner will be looking for definite facts and will be assessing the student's knowledge of some of the statutory duties of the midwife. This type of question is best avoided if the student is not completely sure of her facts as marks are easily lost for inaccurate or missing information.

Sample questions and answers 89

For each section the student should state what the ruling is, its importance and its relevance to the midwife.

SHORT QUESTIONS

Each question accounts for 25 marks.

Q.38 Notification and registration of birth

There are two separate items here which do not often appear together in a short question, therefore the student needs to be aware of the time factor. Both should be described separately, an equal amount of time being given to each element.

(a) Notification of birth

Information given could include:
  (i) who notifies whom and for what reason,
  (ii) time factor,
  (iii) details required on notification form.

(b) Registration of birth
  (i) who registers the birth,
  (ii) where registration takes place,
  (iii) time factor,
  (iv) reasons for registration.

Q.39 Child health clinics

The following information could be included in this answer:

  (i) reasons for having child health clinics,
  (ii) intervals of assessments,
  (iii) who staffs the clinics,
  (iv) where they are normally held.

Q.40 Day care for under-five-year-olds

It is important to note that the student is specifically asked for *day* care, and that there is an age limit of five years. Information included should cover the kind of care provided:

  (i) day nurseries
  (ii) nursery schools
  (iii) playgroups

(iv) crêches
(v) childminders
(vi) daytime nannies

Payment, extent of day care in terms of time and any restrictions on numbers of children cared for could be included if there is time.

Q.41 Fostering
(i) outline what is meant by the term 'fostering',
(ii) selection of foster parents,
(iii) rights of natural parents,
(iv) removal of child from foster care by natural parents,
(v) right to adoption after three years.

Q.42 Early recognition of child abuse
(i) give a definition of what is meant by child abuse,
(ii) how it would be recognized,
   predisposing factors,
   suspicious signs,
   actual abuse,
(iii) what the role of the midwife would be,
(iv) what action should be taken if child abuse is suspected.

Q.43 Unemployed fathers
This short question could be answered in a number of ways. As unemployed fathers are a growing phenomena in the economic climate of today consideration may be given to some of the following:

(i) effects of unemployment on the family as a whole,
(ii) involvement of the father in maternity care as more time is available,
(iii) possibility of the father caring for the baby while the mother goes out to work,
(iv) possible detrimental effects to the family other than financial.

Q.44 Surrogate mothers
This answer could include:

(i) a brief discussion on why this is such an emotive issue,
(ii) the recommendations of the Warnock Report,
(iii) the laws governing surrogacy,
(iv) the psychological effects on both the surrogate and the 'commissioning' mother.

Q.45 *In vitro* fertilization
This could include:

(i) a definition of what is meant by *in vitro* fertilization,
(ii) selection of women,
(iii) counselling,
(iv) moral and ethical issues,
(v) possible effects on maternity and neonatal services.

It would be impossible to mention all the above facets in any depth, therefore either make a brief reference to them or choose one specific aspect to discuss more fully.

Q.46 Asian mother and baby campaign
Topical projects often appear in short questions as a means of identifying the students awareness of current events. The Asian mother and baby campaign is one of these current issues. Included in the discussion should be:

(i) what the campaign is and how it evolved,
(ii) its aims,
(iii) any available results.

Q.47 Financial maternity benefits
It is important to note that the question is about financial benefits and implies those for which the mother gains money. The information required will be quite explicit, therefore if knowledge is limited this question should not be attempted. Information given could include:

(i) which benefits are available,
(ii) how they may be claimed,
(iii) when they may be claimed,
(iv) qualifying conditions,
(v) how long the benefit is paid for, amount.

Q.48 Immunization programmes in the first eighteen months of life

This answer could include:

(i) the reasons for providing an immunization programme,
(ii) the role of the midwife in promoting such a programme,
(iii) the diseases for which immunization is available,
(iv) a brief description of a typical immunization schedule.

Q.49 Threatened abortion

This answer should ideally begin with a definition of *threatened abortion* followed by:

(i) causes of threatened abortion,
(ii) clinical presentation,
(iii) prognosis,
(iv) management (physical and emotional).

Q.50 Hydatidiform mole

A definition of what constitutes a hydatidiform mole is essential here with a description of the features of such a mole (Fig. 4). Further consideration could be given to:

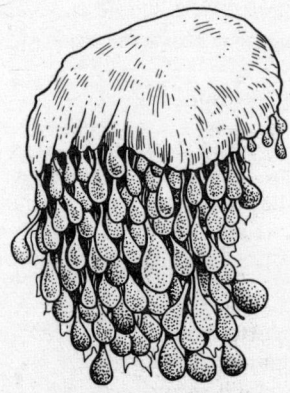

Fig. 4 Hydatidiform mole

Sample questions and answers

(i) clinical picture (uterine changes, effect on mother),
(ii) diagnosis,
(iii) treatment,
(iv) follow-up care,
(v) incidence.

Q.51 The advantages of early uptake of antenatal care
This answer could include:

(i) advantages to mother e.g. meeting 'carers',
(ii) the ability to acquire accurate assessment of gestation,
(iii) the early detection of complications with either mother or fetus,
(iv) the ability to instigate early treatment if complications arise,
(v) the value of early antenatal care in reducing maternal, perinatal and neonatal mortality and morbidity.

Q.52 The risks related to human immunodeficiency virus (HIV/AIDS) in pregnancy
Consider in this answer:

(i) the risk of such a mother to other women and staff,
(ii) the effect of the AIDS virus on the fetus and newborn,
(iii) the psychosocial effects on the mother, her spouse, and her family,
(iv) how HIV is transmitted,
(v) how HIV seropositive women more readily convert to AIDS in pregnancy.

Q.53 Chorionic villus biopsy
This short answer could include:

(i) a description of what chorionic villus biopsy is,
(ii) why it is performed,
(iii) when it is performed,
(iv) possible benefits to the mother over other methods of diagnosing fetal abnormality,
(v) dangers associated with the procedure.

Q.54 Urine testing in pregnancy

This answer should bring out the importance of why we test urine in pregnancy:

(i) what constituents are normally tested for in pregnancy,
(ii) why these specific elements are tested,
(iii) how often urine is tested in pregnancy,
(iv) what abnormal constituents indicate,
(v) a brief outline of what the midwife's role would be if the urine test is abnormal.

Q.55 Asymptomatic bacteriuria

This is a compact short question and should start with a definition of asymptomatic bacteriuria; other information could include:

(i) incidence in pregnancy,
(ii) how the diagnosis is made,
(iii) why it is considered important: that is, what detrimental effects may it have on mother and fetus,
(iv) management – include prophylaxis.

Q.56 Ketonuria

Again this answer should start with a definition of ketonuria; consideration could then be given to:

(i) causes of ketonuria,
(ii) when ketonuria is most likely to develop,
(iii) implications for mother and fetus,
(iv) management.

Q.57 Recognition of impending eclampsia

As with the previous two answers a definition of eclampsia should be given; the remainder of the answer should be devoted to how the student would recognize this emergency situation. The answer could be divided into:

(i) history given by the mother,
(ii) observations of maternal condition by the midwife; it would be relevant to outline dangers to the mother and fetus and possible emergency management.

Sample questions and answers

Q.58 Grande multiparity

Start with a definition of grande multiparity, but keep in mind that the criteria may vary slightly, so try not to be dogmatic:

(i) outline dangers to the mother and fetus and give a brief outline of management,
(ii) be careful not to waste time giving irrelevant information,

This type of short question needs careful thought to enable the student to bring out the most important aspects.

Q.59 Cord presentation

The discerning student will have noticed that the previous four answers all start with a definition of the condition. This is relevant for many short questions and is a useful tactic to remember. This answer should start with a definition of cord presentation and should not be confused with cord prolapse; other information could include:

(i) causative factors associated with cord presentation,
(ii) possible outcomes,
(iii) dangers to the fetus,
(iv) management.

Q.60 Mendelson's syndrome

Define the condition and indicate when it is most likely to occur; further discussion could include:

(i) prevention,
(ii) pathology,
(iii) associated dangers (stress high mortality rate),
(iv) immediate management,
(v) subsequent management if there is time.

Q.61 Antenatal fetal cardiotocography

A short question of this kind can be tackled in several different ways; the examiner would be looking for the following information:

(i) why the procedure may be performed,

(ii) how often it would need to be performed to be of benefit,
   (iii) what is involved,
   (iv) how the results are interpreted and by whom,
   (v) how the information is utilized,
   (vi) role of the midwife.

Q.62 Recognition of the onset of labour
This answer could include:
   (i) how the woman may recognize the onset of labour,
   (ii) how the midwife may recognize the onset of labour, including abdominal and vaginal assessment.
   (iii) how a definite diagnosis of labour is made,
   (iv) implications of diagnosing labour incorrectly.

Q.63 Birth plans
In this answer an explanation should be given of what the student thinks a birth plan is; further consideration could then be given to some of the following aspects:

   (i) how birth plans evolved,
   (ii) value of birth plans in labour,
   (iii) when they should be completed,
   (iv) who should be involved in completion,
   (v) are there any drawbacks to their use,
   (vi) are they inappropriate for some women or should they be available to all.

The amount of time available may not be sufficient to include all the above aspects and the student may need to select those she sees as being most useful.

Q.64 Indications for the midwife to perform an episiotomy
When considering this question it is important to highlight that the question asks for indications for the *midwife* to perform an episiotomy, therefore the answer should omit anything that would come solely within the sphere of the doctor. Information could be given in a list form with a qualifying sentence, divide into:

   (i) maternal indications,
   (ii) fetal indications.

Sample questions and answers

Q.65 Entonox
This short question answer could include:

(i) the composition of Entonox,
(ii) the midwife's rules regarding the administration of Entonox,
(iii) the effect of Entonox on the woman in labour,
(iv) when and how to use Entonox,
(v) storage of Entonox,
(vi) colour of cylinder.

Q.66 Syntometrine
Various drugs often appear in short questions. A similar format could be used to describe important facts for any of them. The ones outlined for Syntometrine would be suitable for many of the other drugs the student is questioned on.

(i) constituents of Syntometrine,
(ii) mode of action,
(iii) when/how it is administered,
(iv) precautions,
(v) contraindications,
(vi) normal dosage.

Q.67 Use of oxytocic drugs in labour
This short question, again dealing with drugs, asks specifically for drug use in labour. In addition to outlining which drugs may fall in to this group the basic information on the pharmacological action should be outlined, as above, with specific reference to its use in labour. Dangers to mother and fetus should also be considered.

Q.68 Moulding of the fetal skull
An explanation should be given of what moulding of the fetal skull is and how and why it occurs (Fig. 5). Normal moulding should be described with an outline of what would be considered abnormal. Dangers of abnormal moulding should be considered along with recognition and reassurance given to the mother.

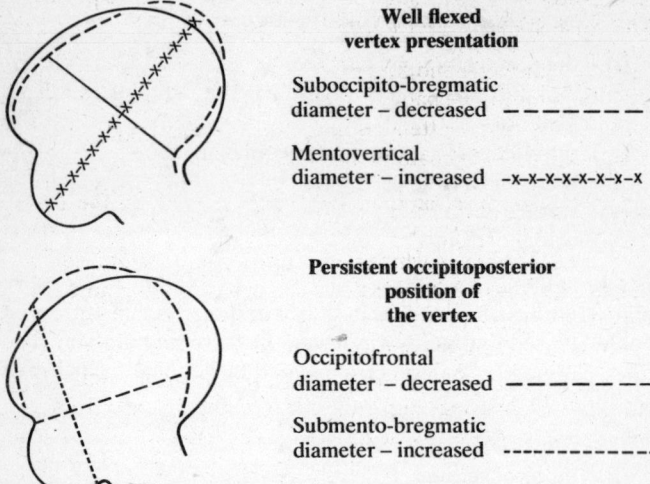

Fig. 5 Moulding of the fetal skull

Q.69 Identification of babies in hospital

This very important procedure has become more topical recently following publicity surrounding babies who have been inadequately identified.

An introduction could include the fact that the majority of babies nowadays are born in hospital therefore adequate identification becomes doubly important, especially with the rapid turnover of mothers and babies because of early transfer. Facts to consider could include:

(i) exactly why babies need to be identified,
(ii) how they are identified,
(iii) how often identification is checked,
(iv) the information required on identification bands,
(v) the procedure should identification labels become loose.

Q.70 Advantages of planned early transfer home

Consideration should be given to defining planned early transfer

Sample questions and answers

home. Note that the question asks for advantages so be positive with your answer, in other words think of:

(i) benefits to the mother,
(ii) benefits for the baby,
(iii) benefits to the attendants,
(iv) benefits to the maternity services as a whole.

Q.71 Opportunities for the education of parents in the postnatal period

This is another topic in which much positive information can be given on the role of the midwife as an educator in the postnatal period.

The question could be answered in broad terms (it is difficult to give much specific information on such a wide topic in a limited space of time) bringing out the opportunity to give information on a one-to-one basis, or as a group after assessing prior knowledge. Consideration may be given to opportunities:

(i) in the hospital setting,
(ii) in the home setting.

Q.72 The effects of prolactin and oxytocin on lactation

This short answer requires fairly specific information (Fig. 6) as there is insufficient time to digress. The answer could include:

(i) where prolactin is produced and its effect on the production of breast milk,
(ii) where oxytocin is produced and its effect on the ejection of milk,
(iii) the value of such knowledge when assisting a mother with breast-feeding,
(iv) effects of inhibition of prolactin and oxytocin on breast milk excretion,
(v) a brief account of any research with which the student is familiar in connection with either of these hormones.

Q.73 Guidance for parents on the feeding of a baby with a cleft lip and palate

This short answer could include:

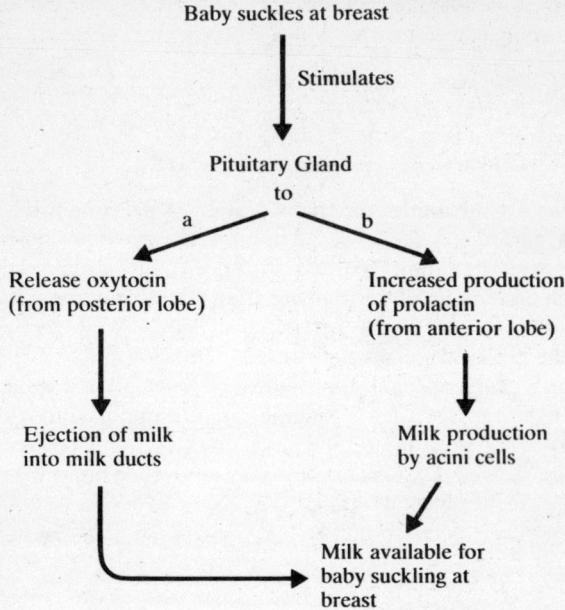

Fig. 6 Diagram to show effects of prolactin and oxytocin on lactation

(i) an explanation to the parents of what cleft lip and palate is,
(ii) reassurance that this problem does not preclude breast-feeding if this was the initial method of choice,
(iii) an account of what measures may be taken to assist with feeding, this latter point could be broken down into breast-feeding and artificial feeding.

Q.74 Tracheo-oesophageal fistula

Included in the answer should be:

(i) a definition of tracheo-oesophageal fistula,
(ii) how it occurs,

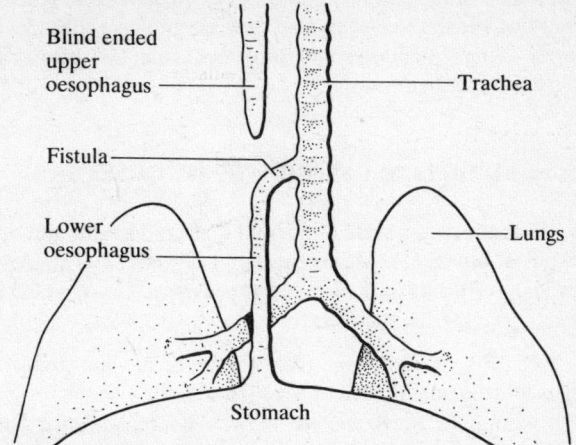

Fig. 7 Diagram to show the commonest form of tracheo-oesophageal fistula

(iii) diagnosis,
(iv) dangers to the baby,
(v) management.

This answer would lend itself well to a diagram (Fig. 7).

Q.75 A midwifery research study/report

Research is being mentioned more and more in examination papers and there is a great deal of encouragement to develop research in midwifery further so that our body of knowledge on which to base practice is enlarged.

If the student chooses to answer this question she should have a specific piece of research in mind. The topic will probably be related to an area in midwifery in which she may have a particular interest, or may have studied in depth for the purpose of a project.

It is important that the student knows the research and acknowledges the author. A little background knowledge as to why the research was carried out would be useful. Essential information would include the findings of the particular research study about which she has chosen to write and its application to midwifery. The student may also like to consider the validity and any limitation of the research.

ADVANCED DIPLOMA IN MIDWIFERY QUESTIONS

Q.76 Pregnancy is a state of normal if altered health and not a condition of illness (R. Methven, 1981). **Discuss this statement and examine critically the rationale and provision of antenatal care.** (*Midwifery paper, March 1987*)

This discussion should range from the medical view that pregnancy is only normal in retrospect to that of the various pressure groups who take the opposite view. The reasons for these diverse views should be explored in detail, with research and statistics quoted, for example, the latest confidential enquiry.

The history of the development of antenatal care and the reduction of mortality rates should also be introduced. A critical analysis should follow which examines social, medical, organizational, and economic reasons that could have contributed to these improvements.

Recent publications that have thrown light on this area of obstetrics could be quoted, such as:

Hall, M., Macintyre, S., and Porter, M. (1985) *Antenatal Care Assessed*, University Press, Aberdeen.
Enkin, M. and Chalmers, I. (1982) *Effectiveness and Satisfaction in Antenatal Care*, Heinemann, London.

In the light of the factors discussed, the argument for selective care for those at risk could follow, including the difficulty in identifying those at risk from complications such as preterm labour.

The site of such provision and the personnel involved can be referred to in relation to the policy document of the Royal College of Midwives – *Towards a Healthy Nation*.

Q.77 Discuss (a) the prevention, (b) early diagnosis of fetal abnormality and (c) the implications for parents.
(*Midwifery paper, March 1986*)

This question consists of three parts, part (a) being *prevention* of fetal abnormality. This needs wide-ranging discussion about the current theories of environmental, biological, and genetic factors and how each of these are being tackled. Comments about regional, national, and international variations should be included before describing local initiatives in the way of preconceptual counselling; discussion should also be included on the fact that those most often at risk are unlikely to use these services, as even when the pregnancy is planned, poor take up of antenatal care is likely. Thought should be given to how this important aspect of health education may be carried out long before pregnancy is possible, possibly in school or through the media.

Part (b) is somewhat non-specific, as 'early' needs special consideration. The ideal time needs to be spelt out, for amniocentesis or chorion villus biopsy in relation to safe termination of pregnancy

This aspect leads into part (c). The implications for the parents are considerable, as before any tests are carried out counselling must include ethical issues arising from their religious, cultural or social background. Any risks involved, and the precise varieties of abnormalities that can be diagnosed, also need to be included. Where a handicapped child may result, parents may wish to talk with either a paediatrician, or other specialist, or other parents who have such a child, so that they may be mentally and emotionally prepared for the birth and subsequent care of the baby. Facilities in the community in the current climate will also need to be included, to demonstrate depth as well as width of knowledge.

Q.78 (a) Explain the physiological factors thought to be responsible for the initiation of labour at term. (b) Discuss possible reasons for preterm labour and the management of this condition.

(*Midwifery paper, November 1987*)

Part (a) asks for a *description* of all the main theories that appear to trigger the initiation of labour. These can be considered under such headings as:

(i) *mechanical* – stretch reflex in the uterus, giving reasons for this hypothesis.

(ii) *hormonal* – the effects of both oestrogen and progesterone on uterine muscle and the cervical tissue – the variation of the balance between them;

the role of prostaglandins;

possible release of oxytocin;

cortisol secretion from fetal adrenals.

Part (b) asks for two items:

(i) *Reasons for preterm labour*; two possible headings could be:

(1) Spontaneous

structural: overstretching as in a multiple pregnancy; trauma to cervix as in late termination of pregnancy;

hormonal: release of prostaglandins in stress or infection;

psychosocial stress;

underprivileged socially, nutritionally, etc.

(2) Induced

maternal reasons such as antepartum haemorrhage, and pre-eclampsia

fetal reasons like intrauterine growth retardation, rhesus incompatibility.

(ii) *Management of this labour*. This will include a discussion of the fetal risks according to the period of gestation suggesting when inhibition of labour will be attempted and by what means. Preparations for the labour should be spelt out including place of delivery and the association with perinatal mortality and morbidity. The management of the labour should be geared towards the special risks which include infection, birth trauma so that mode of delivery should be spelt out, as well as the emotional support the mother will need for this unexpected, as well as possibly dangerous, event.

Q.79 Caesarean section rates vary nationally and internationally. Discuss the factors that may influence these rates.
(*Midwifery paper, November 1987*)

The *initial* part of this question is a statement, but it needs some comments on it. Clarification of the national and international variations are required so that the factors can be identified for the rest of the question.

The *factors* need to be considered globally and not restricted to those relating to obstetrics alone. Possible headings for discussion could be as follows:

(i) Economical factors
 resources,
 geography,
 priorities, political,
 health care system,
 education, degree of expectations of society;
(ii) Individual
 nutritional status,
 stature, etc.;
(iii) Obstetric practice
 intervention,
 interpretation of monitoring procedures,
 litigation concerns,
 place of birth;
(iv) Social pressure
 general public,
 political,
 lay organizations,
 media.

Q.80 **(a) Discuss reasons for postnatal care and its provision. (b) How may this care be improved in the light of current thinking?**
(*Midwifery paper, November 1987*)

This question looks simple, but part (a) needs thinking through carefully, as the description of postnatal care called for in this answer is not straightforward; it involves some political issues as well as midwifery. Few countries have such a care system as in the United Kingdom.

Part (a) considers reasons for postnatal care

(i) Political – it is part of the philosophy of care from the cradle to the grave that formed the basis for the national health service since its inception.
(ii) Maternal vulnerability
physical – genital tract, etc.,
emotional – transition to parenthood.
(iii) Ignorance
nuclear families – social mobility leads to lack of support, education needed in self-care, baby care, family relationships, hygiene, etc.
(iv) Statutory duties
notification, etc.

This is one example in which part (a) may be categorized.

Part (b) considers improvements in this care. A spate of research and reports have emerged in the past few years. Knowledge of the main recommendations must be quoted here and discussed. Titles, authors, and year of publication should be *accurate* if included. Part (b) will take up the major amount of time available.

Q.81 **Describe (a) the characteristics of hypoglycaemia in the first few days of life. (b) How should this condition be managed?**
(*November, 1985*)

In part (a) the characteristics may be subdivided as below:
(i) physical characteristics;

Sample questions and answers

(ii) biochemical characteristics.

In part (b) management headings may be as follows:
(i) prevention of hypoglycaemia by monitoring blood sugar levels on babies at risk;
(ii) early feeding methods, calorific values, etc.;
(iii) monitoring of relevant observations, etc.;
(iv) Treatment:
   careful observation of baby,
   maintenance of blood sugar levels,
   maintenance of body temperature,
   keep parents informed of baby's condition,
   arrange follow-up appointment with paediatrician if blood sugar levels have been very low. Notify health visitor.

Appendix

Past Papers from English National Board, Scottish National Board and Northern Ireland National Board.

THE ENGLISH NATIONAL BOARD FOR NURSING MIDWIFERY AND HEALTH VISITING

MIDWIFERY QUALIFYING EXAMINATION

PAPER 1   3RD NOVEMBER, 1986 FROM 13.30 TO 16.30 HOURS   MARKS

Candidates should answer 3 out of the following 5 questions, allocating approximately 45 minutes to each question.

---

1. Describe the anatomy of the vagina. (30)

   List the indications for a midwife to perform a vaginal examination in labour. (20)

   Discuss the relevance of the information a midwife may obtain when undertaking a vaginal examination on a mother in labour. (50)

                                                                                                                                                                            100

2. Describe the methods of contraception available to parents. (60)

   What factors would you take into consideration when advising a woman and her partner about contraception for the postnatal period? (40)

                                                                                                                                                                            100

3. List the signs of severe neonatal hypothermia. (20)

   How may hypothermia be prevented? (40)

   Describe the management of a baby with severe hypothermia in the first week of life. (40)

                                                                                                                                                                            100

4. A primigravida has fulminating (severe) pre-eclampsia at 38 weeks' gestation.
   How may a midwife recognise this condition? (30)

   What immediate action should she take? (20)

   Outline the subsequent management of this mother by both midwife and obstetrician up until the birth of the baby. (50)

                                                                                                                                                                            100

5. Postnatal care has been described as the "Cinderella of the Maternity Services".
   Describe how midwives can provide first class care and education for mothers and babies during the first 28 days following birth. (100)

Candidates should write on 4 out of the following 8 topics, allocating approximately 10 minutes to each topic.

---

6. (a) Day care for under five year olds. (25)

   (b) Syntometrine. (25)

   (c) Indications for a midwife to perform an episiotomy. (25)

   (d) Grande multiparity. (25)

   (e) Face presentation. (25)

   (f) Infections of the umbilical cord stump. (25)

   (g) Immunisation during the first 18 months of life. (25)

   (h) Ophthalmia neonatorum. (25)

THE ENGLISH NATIONAL BOARD FOR NURSING MIDWIFERY AND HEALTH VISITING

MIDWIFERY QUALIFYING EXAMINATION

PAPER 2   4TH NOVEMBER, 1986 FROM 09.30 TO 12.30 HOURS   MARKS

Candidates should answer 3 out of the following 5 questions, allocating approximately 45 minutes to each question.

---

1. Describe how a midwife would perform an emergency breech delivery in the absence of medical help, giving reasons for her actions. (70)

   Outline the complications of vaginal breech delivery which might affect the newborn baby. (30)

   100

2. With reference to the Report on Confidential Enquiries into Maternal Deaths in England and Wales 1979 - 1981, how may maternal mortality be further reduced? 100

3. What care and advice may be given to a primigravida by the midwife in order to promote and support successful breast feeding:

   a) during pregnancy (40)
   b) in the first 10 days after the birth? (50)

   What help is available to a mother who is breast feeding once she has been discharged from the midwife's care? (10)

   100

4. List the aims of antenatal care. (10)

   Describe in detail how a midwife may achieve these aims. (90)

   100

5. Describe in detail the observations the midwife will make on the mother in the first week following delivery and why these observations are made? 100

Candidates should write on 4 out of the following 8 topics, allocating approximately 10 minutes to each topic.

---

6. (a) Notification and registration of birth. (25)

   (b) Genetic counselling. (25)

   (c) Reasons for inducing labour. (25)

   (d) Unemployed fathers. (25)

   (e) Inhalational analgesia. (25)

   (f) Apgar scoring. (25)

   (g) The pelvic outlet. (25)

   (h) Secondary post partum haemorrhage. (25)

THE ENGLISH NATIONAL BOARD FOR NURSING,
MIDWIFERY AND HEALTH VISITING

MIDWIFERY QUALIFYING EXAMINATION

PAPER 1   12TH JANUARY, 1987 FROM 09.30 TO 12.30 HOURS

Candidates should answer 3 out of the following 5 questions, allocating approximately 45 minutes to each question.   **MARKS**

1. Describe the care a midwife will give to a mother and her baby during the 28 days following delivery.   100

2. A young healthy primigravida is admitted at 42 weeks' gestation to a consultant unit for induction of labour by amniotomy and intravenous oxytocin.
   How should the midwife prepare the parents for these procedures?   (50)

   Describe the care which should be given until labour is established.   (50)

   100

3. Severe fetal abnormality has been diagnosed during the antenatal period.

   (a) How may fetal abnormality be diagnosed in the antenatal period?   (40)

   (b) What care and support can the midwife give to assist parents whose severely abnormal baby is not expected to live more than a few days?   (60)

   100

4. List the causes of neonatal jaundice.   (30)

   Describe the management of severe haemolytic disease in a mature newborn infant.   (60)

   Why has the incidence of severe haemolytic disease declined so significantly over the past 20 years?   (10)

   100

5. Explain the U.K.C.C. Midwives Rules in relation to:-

   (a) Notification of intention to practise.   (25)
   (b) Duty to record the administration of drugs.   (25)
   (c) Duty to keep records.   (25)
   (d) Calling medical assistance in an emergency.   (25)

   100

Candidates should write on 4 out of the following 8 topics, allocating approximately 10 minutes to each topic.

6. (a) Changes in the fetal circulation at birth.   (25)
   (b) Urine testing in pregnancy.   (25)
   (c) Maternal constipation.   (25)
   (d) Threatened abortion.   (25)
   (e) A midwifery research study/report.   (25)
   (f) Causes of psychosexual problems following childbirth.   (25)
   (g) Child health clinics   (25)
   (h) Use of the Pinard's stethoscope.   (25)

THE ENGLISH NATIONAL BOARD FOR NURSING,
MIDWIFERY AND HEALTH VISITING

MIDWIFERY QUALIFYING EXAMINATION

PAPER 2

13TH JANUARY, 1987 FROM 09.30 TO 12.30 HOURS

Candidates should answer 3 out of the following 5 questions, allocating approximately 45 minutes to each question.

MARKS

1. Describe the physiology of the third stage of labour. (30)

   Describe in detail the midwife's management of a newly delivered mother who is bleeding heavily per vaginam following the birth of her baby. (70)

   100

2. It is normal for parents to be particularly anxious during a first pregnancy.

   How may the midwife help to alleviate these anxieties by giving emotional support and antenatal education to both parents? 100

3. Describe the role of the midwife when the mother becomes depressed during the puerperium. 100

4. Describe the vault of the fetal skull. (30)

   How may this knowledge be applied by the midwife during:

   (a) pregnancy (15)
   (b) labour (25)
   (c) the neonatal period? (30)

   100

5. A multipara attends the antenatal clinic at 12 weeks' gestation and is found to have a haemoglobin level of 9.0g/dl.

   (a) List the possible causes of this anaemia. (20)
   (b) What problems are commonly associated with iron deficiency anaemia during pregnancy, labour and the puerperium? (50)
   (c) Outline the possible antenatal management of iron deficiency anaemia. (30)

   100

Candidates should write on 4 out of the following 8 topics, allocating approximately 10 minutes to each topic.

6. (a) Maternity benefits. (25)
   (b) Neonatal hypothermia. (25)
   (c) Sterilization of feeding equipment. (25)
   (d) Asymptomatic bacteriuria. (25)
   (e) Cord presentation. (25)
   (f) Identification of babies in hospital. (25)
   (g) Significance of fetal heart recording in labour. (25)
   (h) Inhalational analgesia. (25)

THE ENGLISH NATIONAL BOARD FOR NURSING,
MIDWIFERY AND HEALTH VISITING

MIDWIFERY QUALIFYING EXAMINATION

PAPER 1 16TH MARCH, 1987 FROM 09.30 TO 12.30 HOURS

Candidates should answer 3 out of the following 5 questions, allocating approximately 45 minutes to each question.

MARKS

1. Describe the factors which may lead to child abuse. (50)

   List the signs of child abuse. (20)

   What action should the midwife take if she suspects a child is being ill-treated or neglected? (30)

   100

2. Following a period of unsatisfactory intra-uterine growth, a baby is born at 38 weeks' gestation with an Apgar score of eight.

   (a) Describe how fetal growth and well-being may have been assessed during pregnancy. (40)

   (b) Discuss the care that may be necessary for the baby during the first week of life. (60)

   100

3. Describe the anatomy of the perineal body. (25)

   Outline how the midwife may prevent or minimise:

   (a) damage to the pelvic floor in labour (35)

   (b) perineal pain during the early postnatal period. (40)

   100

4. Describe the role of the midwife in achieving the aims of antenatal care. 100

5. A mother has had a difficult forceps delivery.

   List the main complications which may occur during the first week. (20)

   Describe the management and the midwifery care of this mother in the first week following delivery. (80)

   100

Candidates should write on 4 out of the following 8 topics, allocating approximately 10 minutes to each topic.

6. (a) Chlamydia. (25)
   (b) Fetal alcohol syndrome. (25)
   (c) Pulmonary embolism. (25)
   (d) The value of research as a basis for practice. (25)
   (e) Succenturiate placenta. (25)
   (f) Meconium stained liquor. (25)
   (g) Spermatozoa. (25)
   (h) Uniovular twins. (25)

THE ENGLISH NATIONAL BOARD FOR NURSING, MIDWIFERY AND HEALTH VISITING

MIDWIFERY QUALIFYING EXAMINATION

PAPER 2 17TH MARCH, 1987 FROM 09.30 TO 12.30 HOURS

Candidates should answer 3 out of the following 5 questions, allocating approximately 45 minutes to each question.

MARKS

1. How would a midwife recognise polyhydramnios during the last trimester of pregnancy? (40)

    List possible causes of polyhydramnios. (30)

    How may the symptoms of this condition be alleviated? (30)
    100

2. How may the midwife help the mother to establish breast feeding successfully when her baby is receiving care in an incubator? 100

3. How may the variations in pelvic size and shape influence the outcomes of labour? 100

4. A mother, following normal delivery of her first baby, is transferred to the postnatal ward.

    (a) Describe the initial assessment of mother and baby by the midwife. (40)

    (b) Outline a plan of care for this mother and her baby for the first 24 hours. (60)
    100

5. Why are some women actively opposed to hospital care and confinement? (40)

    What action should a midwife take when a mother who is considered unsuitable for home delivery insists on having her baby at home? (60)
    100

Candidates should write on 4 out of the following 8 topics, allocating approximately 10 minutes to each topic.

6. (a) Inverted uterus. (25)
    (b) Ergometrine maleate. (25)
    (c) Counselling prior to female sterilization. (25)
    (d) The grieving process. (25)
    (e) Blood pressure recordings during pregnancy. (25)
    (f) Vomiting in the neonate during the first 48 hours following delivery. (25)
    (g) Precipitate delivery. (25)
    (h) Fostering. (25)

**ENGLISH NATIONAL BOARD FOR NURSING,
MIDWIFERY AND HEALTH VISITING**

MIDWIFERY QUALIFYING EXAMINATION

PAPER 1 **11TH MAY, 1987 FROM 09.30 TO 12.30 HOURS**

Candidates should answer 3 out of the following 5 questions, allocating approximately 45 minutes to each question.

MARKS

1. Babies are born in the community and hospital.

   Explain in detail the action the midwife should take in each situation when a baby who has shown fetal distress is born. (100)

2. Explain the dietary advice the midwife may give to pregnant mothers who are:-

   (a) overweight (20)
   (b) experiencing morning sickness (20)
   (c) complaining of heartburn (20)
   (d) suffering from constipation (20)
   (e) vegetarians (20)

   (100)

3. What conditions may predispose to prolapse of the umbilical cord during labour? (20)

   How may cord prolapse be diagnosed during labour? (20)

   Describe the role of the midwife in the management of cord prolapse during labour. (60)

   (100)

4. Health education is an important aspect of the role of the midwife.

   How may she fulfil this duty within the child-bearing population? (100)

5. Physiological changes in the genital tract occur after childbirth.

   (a) Describe these changes. (20)
   (b) Explain their significance. (30)
   (c) How may the midwife recognise deviations from normal during the first 28 days? (50)

   (100)

Candidates should write on 4 out of the following 8 topics, allocating approximately 10 minutes to each topic.

6.
   (a) In vitro fertilization. (25)
   (b) The causes of sore buttocks of the neonate. (25)
   (c) The significance of sickle cell trait. (25)
   (d) Management of postnatal haemorrhoids. (25)
   (e) Safe keeping of controlled drugs on a delivery suite. (25)
   (f) Screening for phenylketonuria. (25)
   (g) Methods of calculating the expected date of confinement. (25)
   (h) Child minders. (25)

THE ENGLISH NATIONAL BOARD FOR NURSING, MIDWIFERY AND HEALTH VISITING

MIDWIFERY QUALIFYING EXAMINATION

PAPER 2 12TH MAY, 1987 FROM 09.30 TO 12.30 HOURS

Candidates should answer 3 out of the following 5 questions, allocating approximately 45 minutes to each question.

MARKS

1. Discuss the value to the mother and her family of continuity of care by the midwife. (100)

2. Labour commences spontaneously at 38 weeks in a multiparous mother with a twin pregnancy, the presentations are cephalic.

   Describe the management of:-

   (a) the second stage of labour (50)
   (b) the third stage of labour. (30)

   List the complications which may occur to the second baby. (20)

   Total: 100

3. Describe the anatomy of the perineal body. (30)

   Explain in detail how the midwife may repair an episiotomy. (70)

   Total: 100

4. Define antepartum haemorrhage. (10)

   The midwife is called to the home of a multiparous mother at 36 weeks gestation who is bleeding per vaginam from a normally situated placental site.

   Describe:-
   (a) the immediate action by the midwife (30)
   (b) the subsequent management and midwifery care for the remainder of the antenatal period. (60)

   Total: 100

5. Congenital abnormality is a major cause of perinatal mortality and morbidity.

   How may the incidence of congenital abnormality be reduced? (100)

Candidates should write on 4 out of the following 8 topics, allocating approximately 10 minutes to each topic

6. (a) The importance of examination of the mother's legs postnatally. (25)
   (b) The role of the National Childbirth Trust. (25)
   (c) Functions of the amniotic fluid. (25)
   (d) Significance to the midwife of the anterior fontanelle. (25)
   (e) State the skin changes occurring during pregnancy. (25)
   (f) The use of prostaglandins in the induction of labour. (25)
   (g) Recognition of normal uterine action in the first stage of labour. (25)
   (h) The effects on the family of sudden infant death syndrome (cot death). (25)

THE ENGLISH NATIONAL BOARD FOR NURSING, MIDWIFERY AND HEALTH VISITING

MIDWIFERY QUALIFYING EXAMINATION

PAPER 1

13TH JULY, 1987 FROM 09.30 TO 12.30 HOURS

Candidates should answer 3 out of the following 5 questions, allocating approximately 45 minutes to each question.

MARKS

1. List the factors predisposing to secondary postpartum haemorrhage. (20)

    Outline the measures which should be taken by a midwife to reduce the risk of this condition occurring. (30)

    In the event of such a haemorrhage occurring at home, what action should be taken by the midwife? (50)

    100

2. What factors should be taken into consideration by the midwife when discussing the choice of contraceptive methods with a recently delivered mother? 100

3. Define Grande Multiparity. (10)

    What potential problems place these women at risk? (30)

    Describe the management of these problems during pregnancy. (60)

    100

4. Describe the care of a pre-term baby born at 34 weeks' gestation. 100

5. A 22 year old primigravida, who is 39 weeks pregnant, is admitted to a consultant unit following spontaneous onset of labour.

    Describe the management of her labour in anticipation of a normal delivery. 100

Candidates should write on 4 out of the following 8 topics, allocating approximately 10 minutes to each topic.

6. (a) The advantages of early uptake of antenatal care. (25)
    (b) Financial maternity benefits. (25)
    (c) The risks related to Human Immuno-Deficiency (AIDS) virus in pregnancy. (25)
    (d) Immunisation programmes in the first 18 months of life. (25)
    (e) The effects of prolactin and oxytocin on lactation. (25)
    (f) Surrogate mothers. (25)
    (g) Entonox. (25)
    (h) Guidance for parents on the feeding of a baby with a cleft lip and palate. (25)

**THE ENGLISH NATIONAL BOARD FOR NURSING,
MIDWIFERY AND HEALTH VISITING**

MIDWIFERY QUALIFYING EXAMINATION

PAPER 2   14TH JULY, 1987 FROM 09.30 TO 12.30 HOURS

Candidates should answer 3 out of the following 5 questions, allocating approximately 45 minutes to each question.

MARKS

1. List the factors which may predispose to deep vein thrombosis in pregnancy, labour and the puerperium. (30)

   Outline the midwife's role in preventing the occurrence of deep vein thrombosis. (70)

   100

2. How may the midwife fulfil her role in promoting and assisting mothers with breast feeding, as well as giving help and support to those who choose to bottle feed their babies? 100

3. What is the effect of pregnancy upon the blood pressure? (10)

   List the possible causes of a raised blood pressure in the last trimester of pregnancy. (20)

   Describe the antenatal management of mild to moderate pre-eclampsia, including support for the whole family. (70)

   100

4. Discuss the wide-ranging role of the midwife within the community. 100

5. How may a midwife recognise a breech presentation? (30)

   Outline the hazards to the baby associated with breech delivery. (30)

   Describe in detail how, in an emergency, a midwife may deliver the aftercoming head of a breech. (40)

   100

Candidates should write on 4 out of the following 8 topics, allocating approximately 10 minutes to each topic.

6. (a) The role of pressure groups in achieving improvement in the maternity services. (25)
    (b) Care of a sutured perineum. (25)
    (c) Ketonuria. (25)
    (d) Birth plans. (25)
    (e) The Local Supervising Authority. (25)
    (f) The Asian Mother and Baby Campaign. (25)
    (g) Involution of the uterus. (25)
    (h) Care of the umbilical cord stump (with reference to research findings). (25)

THE ENGLISH NATIONAL BOARD FOR NURSING,
MIDWIFERY AND HEALTH VISITING

MIDWIFERY QUALIFYING EXAMINATION

PAPER 1   14TH SEPTEMBER, 1987 FROM 09.30 TO 12.30 HOURS

Candidates should answer 3 out of the following 5 questions, allocating approximately 45 minutes to each question.

MARKS

1. How may a midwife recognise postnatal depression? (30)

   List the factors predisposing to depression during the postnatal period. (20)

   What help and support may the midwife give to a depressed mother and her family in the 28 days following delivery? (50)

   100

2. A full term breast fed baby has a small weight loss on the 4th day and a further weight loss on the 6th day of life.

   (a) What information should the midwife obtain to determine possible causes for this weight loss? (50)
   (b) What action should the midwife take? (50)

   100

3. Outline the changes which occur in the uterus during pregnancy. (40)

   What factors influence variations in uterine size during the latter half of pregnancy? (60)

   100

4. Outline the physical and emotional preparation of a mother for elective Caesarean section. (30)

   List the emotional problems which may arise following any Caesarean section. (20)

   Describe briefly the midwife's role in caring for a mother in the first week following Caesarean section. (50)

   100

5. Parentcraft education will need to differ according to various client groups. Discuss this statement. 100

Candidates should write on 4 out of the following 8 topics, allocating approximately 10 minutes to each topic

6. (a) Risks to the second twin during the second stage of labour. (25)
   (b) Colposcopy. (25)
   (c) Chorionic villus biopsy. (25)
   (d) Advantages of caring for healthy pre-term babies in postnatal wards. (25)
   (e) Community Health Councils. (25)
   (f) Examination of the placenta and membranes. (25)
   (g) Tracheo-oesophageal fistula. (25)
   (h) Pentazocine (Fortral) (25)

THE ENGLISH NATIONAL BOARD FOR NURSING,
MIDWIFERY AND HEALTH VISITING

MIDWIFERY QUALIFYING EXAMINATION

PAPER 2   15TH SEPTEMBER, 1987 FROM 09.30 TO 12.30 HOURS

Candidates should answer 3 out of the following 5 questions, allocating approximately 45 minutes to each question.

MARKS

1. Describe in detail the care a primigravida should receive from the midwife when she attends at 38 weeks' gestation for her routine antenatal appointment. — 100

2. Outline the factors which may lead to prolonged labour. (30)

   Describe the role of the midwife in caring for a woman whose labour is prolonged. (70)
   ___
   100

3. Define perinatal mortality. (10)

   List the predisposing factors and main causes of perinatal death. (30)

   How can the midwife use her knowledge and skills to help reduce the incidence of perinatal mortality? (60)
   ___
   100

4. Outline the services available in the community for

   (a) the unsupported working mother with children under five years' of age; (60)
   (b) the family whose new baby has Down's Syndrome. (40)
   ___
   100

5. A multiparous mother at home is found to have a temperature of 39°C on the third postnatal day.

   (a) List the possible causes of the pyrexia. (15)
   (b) What immediate action should the midwife take? (25)
   (c) Describe the management and care of this mother who is diagnosed as having a urinary tract infection. (60)
   ___
   100

Candidates should write on 4 out of the following 8 topics, allocating approximately 10 minutes to each topic.

6. (a) The procedure for the identification of babies whilst in labour ward and postnatal areas. (25)
   (b) Problems of maternal obesity. (25)
   (c) The perineal body. (25)
   (d) Vaginal candidiasis. (25)
   (e) The physiology of lactation. (25)
   (f) The Apgar score. (25)
   (g) The needs of parents whose babies are in a special care baby unit. (25)
   (h) A research study/report concerned with a midwifery aspect of labour. (25)

THE ENGLISH NATIONAL BOARD FOR NURSING,
MIDWIFERY AND HEALTH VISITING

MIDWIFERY QUALIFYING EXAMINATION

PAPER 1   9TH NOVEMBER, 1987 FROM 09.30 TO 12.30 HOURS

Candidates should answer 3 out of the following 5 questions, allocating approximately 45 minutes to each question.

MARKS

1. Describe the vault of the fetal skull. (40)

    How may the midwife use this knowledge

    (a) when making a vaginal examination during labour (30)
    (b) when examining the head of the baby at birth? (30)
    100

2. What range of financial and other benefits may be available to the pregnant woman and her family? 100

3. A mother was unsuccessful in breast feeding her first child. She is pregnant again and very anxious to breast feed this baby.

    What advice, support and encouragement can the midwife give to this mother prior to the birth, and subsequently, so that this time she has more success? 100

4. List the factors which predispose to fetal distress in labour. (10)

    How would the midwife recognise fetal distress during labour? (30)

    Describe how the midwife would resuscitate a baby who fails to breathe at birth. (60)
    100

5. An insulin dependent diabetic is planning to become pregnant.

    What pre-conception advice should she receive? (30)

    Describe her management and care during pregnancy. (70)
    100

Candidates should write on 4 out of the following 8 topics, allocating approximately 10 minutes to each topic.

6.
   (a) The significance of maternal convulsions in pregnancy. (25)
   (b) Indications for rupturing membranes during the first stage of labour. (25)
   (c) Examination of the skin of a healthy newborn baby. (25)
   (d) The importance of the menstrual history at booking. (25)
   (e) Management of secondary postpartum haemorrhage. (25)
   (f) The purpose of birth plans. (25)
   (g) The statutory duties of the midwife during the 28 days following delivery. (25)
   (h) Hypocalcaemia in the newborn. (25)

THE ENGLISH NATIONAL BOARD FOR NURSING,
MIDWIFERY AND HEALTH VISITING

MIDWIFERY QUALIFYING EXAMINATION

PAPER 2   10TH NOVEMBER, 1987 FROM 09.30 TO 12.30 HOURS

Candidates should answer 3 out of the following 5 questions, allocating approximately 45 minutes to each question.

MARKS

1. Pregnancy is a period of change, physical, psychological and emotional.

   How can a midwife assist a mother to adapt to these changes?   100

2. With reference to drug legislation and the United Kingdom Central Council Midwives Rules, describe the midwife's responsibility for supply, storage and administration of drugs.   100

3. A mother is planning to have her second baby at home.

   (a) How may the midwife prepare this family for home confinement?   (40)
   (b) Outline the midwife's management and care of this mother throughout labour.   (60)
   100

4. How may the midwife recognise a twin pregnancy in a mother in labour who has had no antenatal care?   (40)

   What special aspects should the midwife consider when delivering this mother in the absence of medical assistance?   (60)
   100

5. What are the characteristics of a healthy full-term newborn baby?   (40)

   What observations and tests would be carried out within the first 28 days to demonstrate that normal progress is being made?   (60)
   100

Candidates should write on 4 out of the following 8 topics, allocating approximately 10 minutes to each topic.

6. (a) Screening for Rubella during the antenatal period.   (25)
    (b) Ectopic pregnancy.   (25)
    (c) The midwife's management of shoulder dystocia.   (25)
    (d) The use of condoms.   (25)
    (e) Notification and registration of a stillbirth.   (25)
    (f) Procedure for epidural "top-up" by midwives.   (25)
    (g) Imperforate anus.   (25)
    (h) The importance of postnatal exercises.   (25)

THE ENGLISH NATIONAL BOARD FOR NURSING,
MIDWIFERY AND HEALTH VISITING

MIDWIFERY QUALIFYING EXAMINATION

PAPER 1   11TH JANUARY, 1988 FROM 09.30 TO 12.30 HOURS

Candidates should answer 3 out of the following 5 questions, allocating approximately 45 minutes to each question.

MARKS

1. Midwives have a role in antenatal education.

    a) Explain the importance of antenatal education. (40)

    b) Describe the range of opportunities for midwives to educate mothers during pregnancy. (40)

    c) How may the midwife contribute to fulfilling the special needs of mothers for whom English is not their first language? (20)

    100

2. Describe the role of the midwife in supporting and counselling parents and families following stillbirth and neonatal death.   100

3. The midwife sees a multiparous mother at 32 weeks gestation in the community clinic. The mother states that she has had several episodes of painless vaginal bleeding.

    Describe the midwife's action and the subsequent management of this mother.   100

4. Why is a healthy mature newborn baby susceptible to the effects of cold? (20)

    How may neonatal hypothermia be prevented? (20)

    Describe how the midwife may recognise clinical hypothermia. (20)

    What care is required for this condition? (40)

    100

5. Describe the anatomy of the vagina. (30)

    Describe and explain the findings which may be made by a midwife on vaginal examination of a mother during the first, second and third stages of labour. (70)

    100

Candidates should write on 4 out of the following 8 topics, allocating approximately 10 minutes to each topic.

6. (a) Lochia. (25)
    (b) Entonox. (25)
    (c) Policies for the identification of babies in hospital. (25)
    (d) Use of blood transfusion for a child bearing mother. (25)
    (e) Sore nipples. (25)
    (f) Consumption of alcohol in pregnancy. (25)
    (g) Ophthalmia neonatorum. (25)
    (h) Prevention of anaemia during pregnancy. (25)

THE ENGLISH NATIONAL BOARD FOR NURSING, MIDWIFERY AND HEALTH VISITING

MIDWIFERY QUALIFYING EXAMINATION

PAPER 2   12TH JANUARY, 1988 FROM 09.30 TO 12.30 HOURS

Candidates should answer 3 out of the following 5 questions, allocating approximately 45 minutes to each question.

MARKS

1. During the postnatal period, what information should be shared between the midwife in hospital, the midwife in the community and the health visitor so that the mother and baby can receive optimum care? 100

2. A baby born at 30 weeks gestation is being cared for in a neonatal unit.

    a) Describe the appearance of this baby. (20)

    b) What are the particular problems that such a baby might develop? (40)

    c) How would you help the family to be included in the care of their baby? (40)

    100

3. "The use of a planned, individualised system of midwifery care improves the quality of care given to mothers and babies".

    Discuss this statement. 100

4. Outline the physiology of the third stage of labour. (20)

    What are the components of and the action of Syntometrine? (20)

    Describe in detail the midwife's management of the uncomplicated third stage of labour. (60)

    100

5. Describe the effect of pregnancy on the alimentary system. (40)

    What advice should the midwife give in relation to minor disorders affecting this system? (60)

    100

Candidates should write on 4 out of the following 8 topics, allocating approximately 10 minutes to each topic.

6. (a) Glycosuria in pregnancy. (25)
    (b) Protection of a mothers' privacy during labour. (25)
    (c) Abdominal examination of the mother at term. (25)
    (d) The midwife's responsiblity in relation to confidentiality. (25)
    (e) Dietary advice for a mother who is breast feeding. (25)
    (f) Moulding of the fetal skull. (25)
    (g) Management of retention of urine following delivery. (25)
    (h) Day care for children under five years of age. (25)

NATIONAL BOARD FOR NURSING, MIDWIFERY AND HEALTH

VISITING FOR SCOTLAND

MIDWIFERY EXAMINATION

30 JULY 1985

PAPER I

Time allowed ; 2½ hours - 9.30 a.m. to 12 noon

Candidates must answer all four questions.

25 marks are allocated to each question; the numbers in brackets indicate the marks for each part of the question.

1. Felicity is a 37 year old school teacher who is married to an accountant. She is pregnant for the first time and has been very well until now.

   At 35 weeks gestation Felicity develops pre-eclampsia (pregnancy induced hypertension). She is told that monitoring/assessment is to be undertaken.

   1.1 Explain why this is considered necessary and what it involves. (15)

   1.2 Outline the factors which will influence the obstetrician's decision about time and mode of delivery. (7)

   If induction of labour were proposed,

   1.3 Explain to Felicity three reasons for advocating an epidural analgesia during her labour. (3)

2. Ann Jamieson is a 17 year old primigravida at term (40 weeks). Labour began spontaneously ten hours ago but cervical dilatation remains at 4cm.

   2.1 State four conditions which may result in failure to progress in labour. (4)

   2.2 What are the possible effects of failure to progress in labour on both mother and fetus? (6)

   2.3 Outline the nursing and obstetrical management of Ann Jamieson from this time until her baby is delivered. (15)

3. Mrs Bryant had a midcavity forceps delivery for fetal distress. Her baby boy David had severe apnoea (asphyxia neonatorum) and is now in the Neonatal Intensive Care Unit. The prognosis is grave.

   Describe the care that you would give to Mrs Bryant in the postnatal ward to ensure that her emotional needs are met. (25)

4. Outline how the midwife in charge of the ward should respond to the following difficult situations.

   4.1 a three day old breast fed baby will not settle after his feeds (10)
   4.2 a husband arrives with a group of his friends, they are all drunk (5)
   4.3 an episiotomy wound is inflamed and painful (5)
   4.4 a mother decides to discharge herself and her baby at 11 p.m. (5)

NATIONAL BOARD FOR NURSING, MIDWIFERY AND HEALTH

VISITING FOR SCOTLAND

MIDWIFERY EXAMINATION

30 JULY 1985

PAPER II

Time allowed : 2½ hours -1.30 to 4.00 p.m.

Candidates must answer all four questions.

25 marks are allocated to each question; the numbers in brackets indicate the marks for each part of the question.

1. 1.1 State the causes of vomiting in a two day old baby. (5)
   1.2 Describe the investigations and management of this condition. (20)

2. Baby James has just been delivered at term and has a lumbar myelomeningocele.
   2.1 Explain this congenital abnormality using a diagram if desired. Outline the possible effects on the infant. (8)
   2.2 Describe the management of the baby in his first 24 hours following delivery. (12)
   2.3 Outline the implications of this defect in the planning and management of future pregnancies. (5)

3. Discuss the influence of the media on midwifery practice. (25)

4. Mrs Matthew had her second baby four days ago. She and her husband not having used any method of contraception previously now seek advice.
   4.1 State the methods of family planning currently available. (10)
   4.2 Discuss in detail the factors that would influence the advice you would give to them. (15)

NATIONAL BOARD FOR NURSING, MIDWIFERY AND HEALTH

VISITING FOR SCOTLAND

MIDWIFERY EXAMINATION

27 JANUARY 1987

PAPER I

Time allowed: 2½ hours - 9.30 a.m. to 12 noon

Candidates must answer all four questions.

25 marks are allocated to each question; the numbers in brackets indicate the marks for each part of the question.

1. Joan Taylor is a 23 year old married primigravida who is attending the prenatal clinic at 30 weeks gestation. On routine urine testing glycosuria is detected.

1.1 Explain the physiological factors associated with glycosuria in pregnancy. (4)

Following investigation, a diagnosis of diabetes mellitus is made.

1.2 List the fetal and maternal risks associated with diabetes mellitus in pregnancy. (6)
1.3 Describe the subsequent prenatal care required by Joan. (15)

2. Mrs Currie is a 32 year old primigravida who is admitted in labour at term, the following findings are noted:

Height - 1.52 m (5ft)
Bloodgroup - A Rhesus negative
Fetal head - free at the pelvic brim
Membranes - ruptured 24 hours ago.

Explain the potential problems which may arise in her labour and briefly outline the management anticipated for each. (25)

3. 3.1 Describe the process of involution of the uterus. (8)

On abdominal examination, a 35 year old mother is found to have a high uterine fundus on her fourth postnatal day.

3.2 List the possible causes. (5)
3.3 Explain the subsequent management of this mother. (12)

4. Identify the essential elements of instruction and education which should be included in a healthy primiparous patient's postnatal care before she goes home with her normal term baby. (25)

NATIONAL BOARD FOR NURSING, MIDWIFERY AND HEALTH VISITING FOR SCOTLAND

MIDWIFERY EXAMINATION

27 JANUARY 1987

PAPER II

Time allowed: 2½ hours - 1.30 p.m. to 4.00 p.m.

Candidates must answer all four questions.

25 marks are allocated to each question; the numbers in brackets indicate the marks for each part of the question.

The first <u>2 questions</u> in this paper are related to the following.

Jane McGill is an unmarried 18 year old who was discharged from hospital yesterday on her 6th postnatal day following the birth of her first baby Fiona, whom she is bottle feeding.
On visiting Jane you find her living conditions are very poor; the house is cold and damp and Fiona is lying in wet clothes. On examining Fiona you find her temperature is only 32°C.

1. Explain the probable management of Fiona until she is able to maintain her body temperature within normal limits. (25)

2. Jane and Fiona are scheduled to go home again. Outline how the midwife should prepare Jane for this under the following headings:

   2.1 assessment of Jane's knowledge and attitudes (6)
   2.2 specific education and instruction (12)
   2.3 helpful follow up and referral agencies. (7)

3. A full term infant has increasing jaundice on the fourth day of life.

   <u>Explain</u> the

   3.1 investigations made. (10)
   3.2 management required. (15)

4. 4.1 Define perinatal mortality. (2)
   4.2 State the main causes. (3)
   4.3 Describe how the midwife can help to reduce perinatal mortality. (20)

NATIONAL BOARD FOR NURSING, MIDWIFERY AND HEALTH

VISITING FOR SCOTLAND

MIDWIFERY EXAMINATION

28 APRIL 1987

PAPER I

Time allowed: 2½ hours - 9.30 a.m. to 12 noon

Candidates must answer all four questions.

25 marks are allocated to each question; the numbers in brackets indicate the marks for each part of the question.

NB The first three questions are related to the
    following history.

Mrs Flood is a primigravida at 40 weeks gestation.
She has kept well during her pregnancy and has now
been admitted to hospital giving a history of
uterine activity for some hours. Mrs Flood's case
notes are available.

1. 1.1 Outline the information the midwife will
        require from Mrs Flood on admission. (10)
    1.2 An examination per vaginam is carried out to
        assess the progress of Mrs Flood's labour.
        Describe how you would teach a student midwife
        to carry out this procedure and interpret
        the findings.
        (5 marks given for teaching methods) (15)

2. Two hours following the above examination Mrs Flood
    has reached the second stage of labour. Explain the
    midwife's management of the second stage of labour. (25)

3. On the first postnatal day Mrs Flood has an
    eclamptic seizure while her husband is visiting.

    3.1 Explain the midwife's initial management of
        the situation. (10)
    3.2 Outline the management of Mrs Flood for the
        first twenty-four hours following the
        eclamptic seizure. (15)

4. 4.1 Describe the physiological and psychological
        changes which take place during the first 10
        days of the postnatal period. (10)
    4.2 How are these changes assessed? (15)

NATIONAL BOARD FOR NURSING, MIDWIFERY AND HEALTH

VISITING FOR SCOTLAND

MIDWIFERY EXAMINATION

28 APRIL 1987

PAPER II

Time allowed: 2½ hours - 1.30 p.m. to 4.00 p.m.

Candidates must answer all four questions.

25 marks are allocated to each question; the numbers in brackets indicate the marks for each part of the question.

NB ALL questions in this paper should be answered in relation to the following history:

Baby Christopher Jenkins was delivered by mid-cavity forceps at 32 weeks gestation. In good condition at birth, he was transferred to the neonatal unit and is being nursed in an incubator. Christopher weighs 1.8kg and Mrs Jenkins intends to bottle feed her baby.

1. Describe Christopher's physical appearance and behavioural characteristics in comparison with those of the baby in the next incubator who also weighs 1.8kg but was born at 39 weeks gestation. (25)

2. Christopher's progress in the first few days of life has been satisfactory, he is tube fed.

Explain the following:

2.1 The reasons for tube feeding Christopher. (5)
2.2 The technique of passing a nasogastric tube on a preterm baby. (15)
2.3 The potential hazards of tube feeding. (5)

3. A midwife, responding to an apnoea alarm, finds Christopher is apnoeic and deeply cyanosed.

   3.1 Explain the management of this emergency. (20)
   3.2 List 5 possible causes of Christopher's condition. (5)

4. Prolonged separation of mothers and babies is thought to interfere with the normal establishment of parent/baby relationships. Discuss the strategies which can be employed to overcome this problem during Christopher's hospitalisation. (25)

NATIONAL BOARD FOR NURSING, MIDWIFERY AND HEALTH

VISITING FOR SCOTLAND

MIDWIFERY EXAMINATION

28 JULY 1987

PAPER I

Time allowed: 2½ hours - 9.30 a.m. to 12 noon

Candidates must answer all four questions.

25 marks are allocated to each question; the numbers in brackets indicate the marks for each part of the question.

N.B. All <u>four</u> questions are related to the following history.

Joan is 23 years old; her husband Alex is 24 years old. Joan is pregnant for the first time. They are a young couple in good health and have no financial worries. Joan has requested total midwife care.

1. Discuss in detail, the first visit that Joan will make to the midwive's prenatal clinic. (25)

2. Joan is in early labour at term. She is experiencing regular uterine contractions 15 minutes apart; her membranes have not ruptured.

   2.1. What advice would the midwife give to Joan when she telephones the labour ward? (3)
   2.2. Labour is now well established and Joan has been admitted to the labour ward, accompanied by Alex. Describe in detail, the midwifery management of Joan in the first stage of labour. (22)

3. Joan was delivered of baby Stephen 3 minutes ago, the placenta has not been expelled. Joan is now bleeding excessively per vaginam, her general condition remains good.

   3.1. Outline the possible reasons for this haemorrhage. (5)
   3.2. Describe the management of this emergency. (20)

4. Joan has chosen to breastfeed her normal healthy baby, Stephen. You are examining Joan in the postnatal ward on the fourth post-partum day, a student midwife is accompanying you. Describe how you might use this as a learning experience for the student midwife when Joan complains of the following problems.

   4.1. Engorgement of the breasts. (8)
   4.2. Constipation. (5)
   4.3. Feeling faint, tearful and unable to cope with Stephen. (12)

NATIONAL BOARD FOR NURSING, MIDWIFERY AND HEALTH

VISITING FOR SCOTLAND

MIDWIFERY EXAMINATION

28 JULY 1987

PAPER II

Time allowed: 2½ hours - 1.30 p.m. to 4.00 p.m.

Candidates must answer all four questions.

25 marks are allocated to each question; the numbers in brackets indicate the marks for each part of the question.

1. Outline the health education advice which the midwife might give to promote the following for women in her care.

   1.1. adequate fibre in the diet (5)
   1.2. a reduction in cigarette smoking (5)
   1.3. weight control (5)
   1.4. dental care (5)
   1.5. avoidance of self-medication. (5)

2. 2.1. Explain the physiological changes which take place in the human circulatory and respiratory systems at birth. (20)
   2.2. What clinical observations would make a midwife suspect that a newborn infant had a cardiopulmonary abnormality in the first week of life? (5)

3. A newlyborn baby girl has been found abandoned in a telephone box outside a maternity hospital. On admission her weight is 3·2 kg, her temperature 34°C. She is quiet, pale and still. Her extra-uterine age is assessed at 3-4 hours, and her gestational age as "term". Outline the management which will be required in the next 48 hours with regard to the following.

   3.1. achieving and maintaining a normal body temperature. (10)
   3.2. meeting her nutritional needs. (10)
   3.3. discovering her identity. (5)

4. Artificial feeding remains a common method of infant feeding in Britain.

   4.1. Discuss which factors influence the mother to bottle feed her infant. (12)
   4.2. How can a midwife help a mother to become competent in the bottle feeding of her baby? (13)

NATIONAL BOARD FOR NURSING, MIDWIFERY AND HEALTH

VISITING FOR SCOTLAND

MIDWIFERY EXAMINATION

3 NOVEMBER 1987

PAPER I

Time allowed: 2½ hours - 9.30 a.m. to 12 noon

Candidates must answer all four questions.

25 marks are allocated to each question; the numbers in brackets indicate the marks for each part of the question.

NB All questions in this paper are related to the
    following history.

Susan Manning is 25 years old and is pregnant for the
third time. Her sons, Keith and Michael aged four
and two years respectively, are healthy and were
delivered spontaneously at term with no complications.
Susan's husband is an engineer in full time employment.

1. During her first visit to the prenatal clinic
    at 12 weeks gestation, Susan reveals a family
    history of multiple pregnancies.

    1.1 Describe the signs and symptoms which
         would alert the midwife to suspect that
         Susan was expecting twins, and explain
         how a diagnosis of twin pregnancy would
         be confirmed thereafter.   (10)
    1.2 Outline the special aspects of Susan's
         subsequent care during pregnancy.   (15)

2. After an uncomplicated pregnancy and normal
    first stage of labour, Susan has delivered a
    daughter in good condition. The second twin
    is found to be presenting by the breech.
    Vaginal delivery is planned.

    Describe the conduct of the delivery of the
    second twin.   (25)

3. On her 4th postnatal day Susan is found to have a temperature of 38°C. Lochial discharges are scanty. Susan is breast feeding her babies.

   3.1. Explain the investigations of Susan's pyrexia. (12)
   3.2 Indicate the necessary modifications of Susan's postnatal care. (13)

4. Susan and her babies are transferred home on their seventh day. Outline the advice the community midwife may offer to the family to help them:

   4.1 to minimise Susan's tiredness (7)
   4.2 to recognise and cope with sibling rivalry from Keith and Michael (7)
   4.3 with problems of differentiating between the identical twin girls, thus enabling them to develop as individuals. (11)

NATIONAL BOARD FOR NURSING, MIDWIFERY AND HEALTH

VISITING FOR SCOTLAND

MIDWIFERY EXAMINATION

3 NOVEMBER 1987

PAPER II

Time allowed: 2½ hours - 1.30 p.m. to 4.00 p.m.

Candidates must answer all four questions.

The numbers in brackets indicate the marks for each part of the question.

NB   All questions in this paper are related to the
     following history

Robert is the first child of Tom and Mary Rankin, both
of whom are 35 years old. Mary has had four previous
unsuccessful pregnancies. At 39 weeks gestation
spontaneous labour began and fetal distress occurred.
An emergency caesarean section was carried out.

1. Robert who weighs 3.9 kg, was asphyxiated at
    birth, his Apgar score was 5 at 5 minutes. The
    amniotic fluid was meconium stained.

    1.1 Justify Robert's transfer to the neonatal
         unit following resuscitation. (5)
    1.2 Explain his care in the first 24 hours
         after the admission procedure is
         completed. (25)

                                                (30)

2. After 48 hours Robert is transferred to the
    postnatal ward. Mary, who had initially
    indicated that she wished to bottle feed her
    son, now says that she wants to breast feed
    him.

    Describe :-

    2.1 the physiology of lactation. (8)
    2.2 how you would assist Mary to put Robert
         to the breast for the first time. (5)
    2.3 the information which you would give to
         Mary about breast feeding. (12)

3. Although Mary and Tom would like to have another baby they would like to wait until their son is about two years old.

   Taking account of the information given about this family, explain the advice you would offer Mary and Tom regarding :-

3.1	family spacing	(5)
3.2	suitable contraceptive methods.	(15)
		(20)

4. Outline the information which you would give to Mary when she asks about the following :-

4.1	neonatal hypothermia	(5)
4.2	weaning	(5)
4.3	immunisation	(5)
4.4	child health clinic	(5)
4.5	child benefit.	(5)

THE NATIONAL BOARD FOR NURSING, MIDWIFERY AND HEALTH VISITING FOR NORTHERN IRELAND

FINAL EXAMINATION FOR ADMISSION TO PART 10 OF THE REGISTER - MIDWIFERY

THURSDAY 24TH JANUARY 1985

FIRST PAPER

Time allowed 2 hours - 9.15 a.m. to 11.15 a.m.

IMPORTANT Read the questions carefully and answer only what is asked as no credit will be given for irrelevant matter.

NOTE Candidates should attempt ALL QUESTIONS.

		Marks
1. (a)	List the temporary structures in the fetal circulation.	5
(b)	Describe the changes which occur in the circulation at birth.	20
		25

2. Explain the effects of:-

(i)	the gonadotrophic hormones on the ovary	12
(ii)	the ovarian hormones on the endometrium	13
		25

149

	Marks

3. Describe the factors which may contribute to perineal lacerations. — 25

4. (a) Draw and label a diagram of the vagina and its anatomical relationships. — 8

   (b) List the indications for vaginal examination in normal labour. — 8

   (c) Describe the information which can be obtained about the cervix from such an examination. — 9

   Total: 25

5. (a) Define the post-natal period. — 3

   (b) Describe the changes which occur duing the puerperium in relation to the following:-

   (i) the uterus — 11
   (ii) the blood and blood vessels — 11

   Total: 25

6. Explain, with the aid of a diagram, the physiology of lactation. — 25

7. Explain why the following conditions may occur in a neonate:-

   (i) hypernatraemia — 12
   (ii) hypothermia — 13

   Total: 25

8. Describe the statutory rules for midwives which apply to each of the following:-

   (i) supervision of midwives — 5
   (ii) suspension from practice — 5
   (iii) record keeping — 5
   (iv) administration of inhalational analgesia — 10

   Total: 25

THE NATIONAL BOARD FOR NURSING, MIDWIFERY AND HEALTH VISITING FOR NORTHERN IRELAND

FINAL EXAMINATION FOR ADMISSION TO PART 10 OF THE REGISTER - MIDWIFERY

SECOND PAPER

Friday 25th January 1985

Time allowed 3 hours - 9.15 a.m. to 12.15 p.m.

IMPORTANT Read the questions <u>carefully</u> and answer only what is asked as no credit will be given for irrelevant matter.

NOTE Candidates should attempt FIVE questions:-
The <u>one</u> in Section A, <u>three</u> from Section B, and <u>one</u> from Section C.

SECTION A

Marks

1. A twenty-six year old primigravida at twenty-eight weeks gestation is suspected of having a twin pregnancy.

    (a) Describe the midwife's role in helping to diagnose twins. — 30

    The diagnosis is confirmed.

    (b) Describe the subsequent care of this woman in relation to:-

    (i) prevention of premature labour — 20
    (ii) prevention of anaemia — 20

    (c) Describe the advice and guidance this woman should receive with regard to financial benefits. — 30

    100

SECTION B

2. (a) Describe the management of a patient during the third stage of labour in relation to:-

    (i) separation of the placenta — 20
    (ii) delivery of the placenta and membrane by the modified Brandt-Andrews manoeuvre — 20
    (iii) use of oxytocic medicines — 20

    (b) Describe the immediate care which should be given to a patient who develops a primary post-partum haemorrhage in the third stage of labour. — 40

    100

SECTION B CONT'D

Marks

3. A mother with eclampsia is to be transferred to hospital from home.

   (a) Describe the responsibilities of the midwife in relation to the transfer.   25

   (b) Describe the midwifery management of this patient prior to delivery in relation to:-

(i)	safety	25
(ii)	observations and their significance	30
(iii)	medications which may be prescribed	20
		100

4. Describe the advice midwives should give to mothers about to be transferred home in relation to:-

(i)	immunisation and vaccination	25
(ii)	parent/child relationships	25
(iii)	family planning services	25
(iv)	the importance of the post-natal examination at the end of the puerperium.	25
		100

5. Describe the management of the following which may occur in the post-natal period:-

(i)	mastitis	30
(ii)	puerperal depression	35
(iii)	deep venous thrombosis	35
		100

SECTION C

Marks

6. An infant has failed to gain weight by the tenth post-natal day.

   (a) Describe the management of this infant in relation to:-

   (i) observations and their significance   25
   (ii) investigations   25

   No pathological cause has been identified.

   (b) Describe:-

   (i) a suitable artificial feeding regime for this infant   25
   (ii) how the mother may be helped to care for the infant following transfer home.   25

                                                                                                                                     100

7. Describe:-

   (i) the measures taken to reduce the incidence of infection in a maternity hospital   50

   (ii) the responsibilities of a midwife when a mother and baby are to be transferred to the care of a Community Midwife.   50

                                                                                                                                     100

THE NATIONAL BOARD FOR NURSING, MIDWIFERY AND HEALTH VISITING FOR NORTHERN IRELAND

FINAL EXAMINATION FOR ADMISSION TO PART 10 OF THE REGISTER - MIDWIFERY

FIRST PAPER

Thursday 25th April 1985

Time allowed 2 hours - 9.15 a.m. to 11.15 a.m.

IMPORTANT   Read the questions carefully and answer only what is asked as no credit will be given for irrelevant matter.

NOTE   Candidates should attempt ALL questions.

	Marks

1. Explain why the following disorders may occur during pregnancy:-

   (i) varicose veins — 7
   (ii) backache — 6
   (iii) fainting — 6
   (iv) heart burn — 6

   Total: 25

2. (a) Draw and label a diagram of the fetal skull. — 8

   (b) Explain how cephalo-pelvic disproportion may be diagnosed in the pre-natal period. — 10

   (c) Describe how cephalo-pelvic disproportion may affect the mode of delivery. — 7

   Total: 25

	Marks

3. (a) List the clinical features of fetal hypoxia in labour. — 9

   (b) List the observations which should be made during labour to assess:-

   (i) maternal condition — 6
   (ii) fetal condition — 4
   (iii) progress of labour — 6

   Total: 25

4. (a) Define the third stage of labour. — 5

   (b) Describe the signs of separation and descent of the placenta. — 5

   (c) Describe the delivery of the placenta and membranes by controlled cord traction. — 15

   Total: 25

5. (a) Define secondary post-partum haemorrhage. — 5

   (b) List the factors which may predispose to the onset of urinary tract infection after delivery. — 8

   (c) List the investigations which may be made on a patient who has a raised temperature on the third day of the puerperium. — 12

   Total: 25

6. Explain the importance of the observations of a mother during the post-natal period in relation to:-

   (i) involution of the uterus — 8
   (ii) urinary output — 8
   (iii) emotional state — 9

   Total: 25

7. (a) Explain why hypoglycaemia may occur in the newborn. — 17

   (b) Describe how this condition may be diagnosed. — 8

   Total: 25

8. Compare and contrast the clinical features of a pre-term and a "small for gestational age" infant. — 25

155

THE NATIONAL BOARD FOR NURSING, MIDWIFERY AND HEALTH VISITING FOR NORTHERN IRELAND

FINAL EXAMINATION FOR ADMISSION TO PART 10 OF THE REGISTER - MIDWIFERY

SECOND PAPER

Friday 26th April 1985

Time allowed 3 hours - 9.15 a.m. to 12.15 p.m.

IMPORTANT Read the questions carefully and answer only what is asked as no credit will be given for irrelevant matter.

NOTE Candidates should attempt **FIVE** questions:-

The one in Section A, three from Section B, and one from Section C.

SECTION A

Marks

1. A primigravida attends the ante-natal clinic for the first visit at the tenth week of her pregnancy.

    (a) Describe the advice which should be given to this woman during the pregnancy in relation to:-

(i)	diet	15
(ii)	alcohol consumption	15
(iii)	cigarette smoking	10
(iv)	anxiety about labour	25

    (b) Explain the significance of the following during pregnancy:-

(i)	blood tests	20
(ii)	urine tests	15
		100

SECTION B

2. A multiparous woman at thirty-eight weeks gestation is admitted in labour with a breech presentation.

    (a) Describe the care of this patient on admission in relation to:-

(i)	observations	20
(ii)	abdominal examination	20
(iii)	vaginal examination	20

    (b) Describe how the midwife may minimize the risks during delivery for:-

(i)	the mother	20
(ii)	the infant	20
		100

SECTION B CONT'D

	Marks

3. (a) Describe the management of a patient during the third stage of labour in relation to:-

    (i) separation of the placenta — 10
    (ii) delivery of the placenta and membranes by the modified Brandt-Andrews manoeuvre — 25
    (iii) use of oxytocic medicines — 25

  (b) Describe the immediate care which should be given to a patient who develops a primary post-partum haemorrhage in the third stage of labour. — 40

                                                                                                  100

4. A primipara, following a normal delivery, is to breast feed her baby.

  (a) Describe the midwife's role in relation to:-

    (i) minimizing the mother's anxiety — 30
    (ii) care of the breasts — 15
    (iii) the technique and frequency of feeding — 25

  (b) Describe how the midwife may help the mother overcome the following problems which may be encountered in breast feeding:-

    (i) cracked nipples — 15
    (ii) insufficient lactation — 15

                                                                                                  100

5. A primipara has had a forceps delivery.

  (a) Describe the midwifery management of this woman in hospital in relation to:-

    (i) retention of urine — 25
    (ii) oedema and bruising of the perineum — 25
    (iii) rest and sleep — 25

  (b) Describe how the risks of infection may be minimized in the post-natal ward. — 25

                                                                                                  100

SECTION C

Marks

6. Describe the role of the midwife in relation to the following:-

    (i) the care of an infant having phototherapy   35

    (ii) the immediate care of an infant who develops a convulsion   35

    (iii) a mother who is distressed at being unable to breast feed her sick infant.   30

      100

7. Describe the responsibilities of the midwife in charge of a ward in relation to:-

    (i) administration of medicines   25

    (ii) transfer of mother and baby to the care of the Community Midwife   25

    (iii) communication within the ward   25

    (iv) improving standards of patient care   25

      100

THE NATIONAL BOARD FOR NURSING, MIDWIFERY AND HEALTH VISITING FOR NORTHERN IRELAND

FINAL EXAMINATION FOR ADMISSION TO PART 10 OF THE REGISTER - MIDWIFERY

FIRST PAPER

THURSDAY 25TH JULY 1985

Time allowed 2 hours 9.15 a.m. to 11.15 a.m.

IMPORTANT Read the questions **carefully** and **answer only what is asked** as no credit will be given for irrelevant matter.

NOTE Candidates should attempt ALL questions.

	Marks

1. (a) Draw and label diagrams of the pelvic brim and outlet to show:-

    (i) the shape of the gynaecoid pelvis — 5
    (ii) the anterio-posterior diameters — 5
    (iii) the oblique diameters — 5
    (iv) the transverse diameters — 5

   (b) Explain the term engagement of the fetal head. — 5

   Total: 25

2. Explain the use of the following methods of assessing intra-uterine fetal well-being:-

    (i) ante-natal cardiotocography — 8
    (ii) serial oestriol estimations — 8
    (iii) serial ultrasanography — 9

   Total: 25

  Marks

3. (a) Explain the following in relation to the fetus:-

        (i)   position   6
        (ii) attitude of the head   6

    (b) Explain moulding of the skull which occurs as a result of:-

        (i)   occipito anterior position   6
        (ii) occipito posterior position   7
                                                                      ──
                                                                      25

4. (a) List the methods of pain relief in labour.   9

    (b) Define epidural analgesia.   4

    (c) Explain why hypotension may occur during epidural analgesia. 12
                                                                      ──
                                                                      25

5. (a) Explain the physiology of lactation under the following
        headings:-

        (i)   production of milk   4
        (ii) flow of milk   4
        (iii) withdrawal of milk   4
        (iv) maintenance of supply   4

    (b) List the advantages of breast feeding to the:-

        (i)   mother   4
        (ii) baby   5
                                                                      ──
                                                                      25

6. (a) Define post-partum haemorrhage.   5

    (b) List the possible causes of this condition.   10

    (c) Describe the use of oxytocin as a prophylactic measure.   10
                                                                      ──
                                                                      25

7. (a) Explain the process of rhesus immunisation in the rhesus
        negative pregnant woman.   7

    (b) Describe the use of the following:-

        (i)   Coomb's test   5
        (ii) Kleihauer test   5
        (iii) Rh anti-D immunoglobulin   8
                                                                      ──
                                                                      25

	Marks
8. (a) Define non-accidental injury.	4
(b) List the factors which predispose to non-accidental injury.	6
(c) Describe how the midwife may contribute to the prevention of non-accidental injury through pre-natal education.	15
	25

THE NATIONAL BOARD FOR NURSING, MIDWIFERY AND HEALTH VISITING FOR NORTHERN IRELAND

FINAL EXAMINATION FOR ADMISSION TO PART 10 OF THE REGISTER - MIDWIFERY

SECOND PAPER

FRIDAY 26TH JULY 1985

Time allowed 3 hours - 9.15 a.m. to 12.15 p.m.

IMPORTANT   Read the questions carefully and answer only what is asked as no credit will be given for irrelevant matter.

NOTE   Candidates should attempt FIVE questions:-
The one in Section A, three from Section B,
and one from Section C.

SECTION A

Marks

1. A multipara at ten weeks gestation is attending the pre-natal clinic for the first time.

   Describe the significance of the following in relation to this woman:-

(i)	social history	25
(ii)	medical history	25
(iii)	obstetric history	25
(iv)	history of present pregnancy	25
		100

SECTION B

2. A multiparous woman with severe Cardiac Disease is transferred to the Delivery Suite in established labour at 39 weeks gestation.

   Discuss the management of this patient under the following headings:-

(i)	observations and their significance	40
(ii)	relief of pain	40
(iii)	preparation for delivery	20
		100

SECTION B CONT'D

Marks

3. A patient with severe pre-eclampsia is admitted in labour at thirty-six weeks gestation.

   (a) Describe the management of this patient under the following headings:-

   (i) assessment of the patient's condition on admission 25
   (ii) medicines which may be prescribed, stating their action, dose and side effects 25
   (iii) on-going observations and their significance 25

   (b) Describe the immediate care of the baby following delivery. 25

   100

4. A primipara has a third degree tear following a difficult delivery.

   (a) Explain the significance of the examination which should be carried out on this woman. 30

   (b) Describe the management of this patient for the first five days following delivery in relation to:-

   (i) the third degree tear of the perineum 25
   (ii) urinary complications which may occur 25
   (iii) emotional support 20

   100

5. A twenty year old woman develops a puerperal sepsis on the sixth day following an uncomplicated delivery.

   Describe the midwifery management of this patient in relation to:-

   (i) investigations 30
   (ii) minimizing the risk of the spread of infection 30
   (iii) nutrition 20
   (iv) reducing temperature 20

   100

	SECTION C	Marks

6. Describe the responsibilities of the midwife in charge of a ward in relation to:-

   (i)   administration of medicines — 25

   (ii) transfer of mother and baby to the care of the Community Midwife — 25

   (iii) communication within the ward — 25

   (iv) improving standards of patient care — 25

   Total: 100

7. A baby develops convulsions forty-eight hours after birth.

   (a) Explain the significance of the observations which should be made on this infant. — 30

   (b) Describe the care of this infant:-

   (i) pending the arrival of the doctor — 20
   (ii) during the subsequent forty-eight hours — 25

   (c) Describe how the midwife may help to minimize the parents' anxiety. — 25

   Total: 100

THE NATIONAL BOARD FOR NURSING, MIDWIFERY AND HEALTH VISITING FOR NORTHERN IRELAND

FINAL EXAMINATION FOR ADMISSION TO PART 10 OF THE REGISTER - MIDWIFERY

FIRST PAPER

THURSDAY 24TH OCTOBER 1985

Time allowed 2 hours - 9.15 a.m. to 11.15 a.m.

IMPORTANT Read the questions carefully and answer only what is asked as no credit will be given for irrelevant matter.

NOTE Candidates should attempt ALL questions.

		Marks
1. (a)	Draw and label a diagram to illustrate the landmarks of the gynacoid pelvis.	10
(b)	Explain the special features of a gynacoid pelvis.	15
		25
2. (a)	List the functions of the placenta.	10
(b)	Describe how placental function may be assessed.	15
		25

  Marks

3. (a) Draw and label a diagram of the:-

    (i) superficial muscles of the pelvic floor   7
    (ii) deep muscles of the pelvic floor   7

    (b) Discuss the indications for episiotomy.   11
                                                                     ──
                                                                     25

4. Describe the development of the chorionic villi from the
    trophoblastic layer of the blastocyst.   25

5. (a) Describe the physiology of the uterus in the puerperium.   15

    (b) Explain the clinical features of sub-involution of the
        uterus.   10
                                                                     ──
                                                                     25

6. (a) Explain the use of the Apgar Score at birth.   10

    (b) Describe the principles of resuscitation of an infant
        at birth.   15
                                                                     ──
                                                                     25

7. (a) Draw and label a diagram of the internal structures of
        the fetal skull.   10

    (b) Describe the factors which may contribute to intracranial
        injury in the newborn.   15
                                                                     ──
                                                                     25

8. An unmarried primipara has decided to keep her baby.

    List the resources available to her under the following headings:-

    (i) financial   12
    (ii) social   13
                                                                     ──
                                                                     25

THE NATIONAL BOARD FOR NURSING, MIDWIFERY AND HEALTH VISITING FOR NORTHERN IRELAND

FINAL EXAMINATION FOR ADMISSION TO PART 10 OF THE REGISTER - MIDWIFERY

SECOND PAPER

FRIDAY 25TH OCTOBER 1985

Time allowed 3 hours - 9.15 a.m. to 12.15 p.m.

IMPORTANT   Read the questions carefully and answer only what is asked as no credit will be given for irrelevant matter.

NOTE   Candidates should attempt FIVE questions:-

The one in Section A, three from Section B, and one from Section C.

SECTION A

Marks

1. A woman is admitted to hospital at thirty-six weeks gestation with a history of bleeding per vaginam.

   (a) Describe the history specific to the bleeding which the midwife should take.   25

   Two days after admission, this patient has a severe haemorrhage per vaginam.

   (b) Describe the management of this patient:-

   (i) in the period immediately following the haemorrhage   35
   (ii) in the subsequent period prior to delivery by Caesarean section.   40

   100

SECTION B

2. (a) Compare and contrast the findings on abdominal examination between vertex and breech presentations.   30

   A multiparous patient is admitted to hospital in advanced labour with a flexed breech presentation.

   (b) Describe the delivery of the infant by the midwife.   40

   (c) Describe the possible risks during delivery for:-

   (i) the mother   10
   (ii) the infant   20

   100

	SECTION B CONT'D	Marks

3. (a) Describe the care during labour of a primigravida at term in relation to:-

    (i) routine observations and their significance   25
    (ii) pain relief   35

   (b) Describe the care of her baby in the hour following delivery in relation to:-

    (i) respiratory function   20
    (ii) body temperature   20
                            100

4. Describe how the Community Midwife may manage in the following situations:-

   (i) a mother complains of persistent red lochia on the sixth post-natal day   25

   (ii) a mother whose sleep pattern has been disturbed since the birth of her baby   25

   (iii) a mother who is concerned about becoming pregnant again too soon   25

   (iv) a mother is worried about a persistent discharge from her infant's eyes.   25
                            100

5. Describe the care required when the following complications occur in the post-natal period:-

   (i) a multiparous woman develops deep venous thrombosis on the fifth post-natal day   30

   (ii) a twenty-two year old woman has a painful perineum and haemorrhoids   25

   (iii) a forty year old multipara has stress incontinence   20

   (iv) a twenty-six year old primipara has "fourth day blues".   25
                            100

	SECTION C	Marks

6. (a) Describe the examination of a baby during the first hour of life.   40

    Following examination, an infant is discovered to have a cleft lip and palate.

   (b) Describe the midwife's role in relation to:-

      (i)   psychological support for the parents   20
      (ii) feeding   20
      (iii) developing a good parent/child relationship   20

                                                                                             100

7. Describe the management of the following:-

   (i)   oral thrush in a four day old infant   25
   (ii) inflammation of the umbilicus in a three day old infant   25
   (iii) excoriation of the buttocks in a ten day old infant   25
   (iv) jaundice in a three day old infant   25

                                                                                             100

THE NATIONAL BOARD FOR NURSING, MIDWIFERY AND HEALTH VISITING FOR NORTHERN IRELAND

FINAL EXAMINATION FOR ADMISSION TO PART 10 OF THE REGISTER - MIDWIFERY

FIRST PAPER

THURSDAY 23RD JANUARY 1986

Time allowed 2 hours - 9.15 a.m. to 11.15 a.m.

IMPORTANT — Read the questions carefully and answer only what is asked as no credit will be given for irrelevant matter.

NOTE — Candidates should attempt ALL questions.

		Marks
1. (a)	Describe a chorionic villus.	10
(b)	List the factors which may reduce the supply of oxygen to the fetus before birth.	15
		25
2. (a)	Draw and label a diagram of the pelvic brim.	9
(b)	Describe the diameters of the pelvic brim and state their average measurements.	12
(c)	List the methods of assessing the size and shape of the pelvic brim.	4
		25

	Marks

3. Describe the possible effects of occipito-posterior position during:-

    (i) the first stage of labour   12

    (ii) the second stage of labour   13

                                                                                      25

4. Distinguish between the following:-

    (i)   false and true labour   10

    (ii)   presentation and position   8

    (iii) retraction ring and Bandl's ring   7

                                                                                      25

5. (a) Draw and label a diagram of the fetal circulation.   15

   (b) List the changes which occur in the circulation at birth.   10

                                                                                      25

6. (a) Explain the physiology of lactation under the following headings:-

       (i)   production of breast milk   7

       (ii)   flow of breast milk   7

       (iii) withdrawal of breast milk   7

   (b) List four factors which may inhibit successful lactation.   4

                                                                                      25

7. (a) List five possible side effects of the contraceptive pill.   5

   (b) Discuss four factors which should be considered when giving advice to a woman about choosing a contraceptive method and explain the significance of the advice given.   20

                                                                                     25

8. Explain how the following may occur in the neonate:-

    (i)   physiological jaundice   7

    (ii)   kernicterus   6

    (iii) talipes   6

    (iv)   oral thrush   6

                                                                                      25

THE NATIONAL BOARD FOR NURSING, MIDWIFERY AND HEALTH VISITING FOR NORTHERN IRELAND

FINAL EXAMINATION FOR ADMISSION TO PART 10 OF THE REGISTER - MIDWIFERY

SECOND PAPER

FRIDAY 24TH JANUARY 1986

Time allowed 3 hours - 9.15 a.m. to 12.15 p.m.

IMPORTANT   Read the questions carefully and answer only what is asked as no credit will be given for irrelevant matter.

NOTE   Candidates should attempt **FIVE** questions:-
The one in Section A, three from Section B and one from Section C.

SECTION A

Marks

1. A thirty-five year old primigravida at 37 weeks gestation attends the ante-natal clinic:-

    (a) Describe the advice she should be given by the midwife in relation to:-

(i)	breast feeding	35
(ii)	the onset of labour	35

    (b) Discuss the factors which should be considered in determining the mode of delivery in this case.   30

    100

SECTION B

2. A primigravida is admitted at 32 weeks gestation in established labour.

    (a) Describe the management of labour in relation to:-

(i)	the relief of pain	20
(ii)	observations of fetal well-being	20
(iii)	preparations for the reception of a premature infant	20

    (b) Explain the immediate care of the infant with particular reference to establishing and maintaining respiration.   40

    100

SECTION B CONT'D

Marks

3. A primigravida at 42 weeks gestation is to have labour induced.

   (a) Explain the reasons why labour should be induced at this time.　　20

   Labour is induced by amniotomy followed by Syntocinon infusion.

   (b) Describe the management of the first stage of labour under the following headings:-

(i)	observations and their significance	40
(ii)	nursing care	40

   　　　　　　　　　　　　　　　　　　　　　　　100

4. (a) Describe the care of a mother in the first ten days of the puerperium under the following headings:-

(i)	daily examination	30
(ii)	nutrition	20
(iii)	rest and exercise	20

   (b) Explain how the midwife may contribute to the promotion of a good parent/child relationship.　　30

   　　　　　　　　　　　　　　　　　　　　　　　100

5. A multiparous woman has a post-partum haemorrhage at home on the tenth post-natal day.

   (a) Describe the care which should be given by the midwife in relation to:-

(i)	the control of the haemorrhage	30
(ii)	the immediate needs of the family	20

   (b) Explain the significance of the following in the management of this patient on admission to hospital:-

(i)	observations	25
(ii)	investigations	25

   　　　　　　　　　　　　　　　　　　　　　　　100

173

SECTION C

		Marks
6. A four day old infant becomes listless and refuses to feed.

    (a) Describe the observations which should be made. — 25

    (b) Explain the significance of the investigations which should be carried out. — 25

This infant is diagnosed as having cerebral damage.

    (c) Describe the care of this infant in relation to:-

        (i) nutrition — 25
        (ii) temperature control — 25

    Total: 100

7. (a) Discuss the causes of perinatal mortality in Northern Ireland. — 35

    (b) Discuss the midwife's role in relation to the reduction of the perinatal mortality rate under the following headings:-

        (i) genetic counselling and screening — 20
        (ii) research — 20
        (iii) health education — 25

    Total: 100